BAGUA AND TAI CHI

Other Books by Bruce Frantzis

Tao of Letting Go:
Meditation for Modern Living

Relaxing into Your Being (Taoist Meditation, Volume 1):
Chi, Breathing and Dissolving Inner Pain

The Great Stillness (Taoist Meditation, Volume 2):
Body Awareness, Moving Meditation and Sex Qigong

Chi Revolution:
Harness the Healing Power of Your Life Force

Dragon and Tiger Medical Qigong:
Health and Energy in Seven Simple Movements

Opening the Energy Gates of Your Body:
Qigong for Lifelong Health

The Power of Internal Martial Arts and Chi:
Combat and Energy Secrets of Bagua, Tai Chi and Hsing-I

Tai Chi: Health for Life:
Why It Works for Health, Stress Relief and Longevity

BAGUA AND TAI CHI

Exploring the Potential of Chi,
Martial Arts, Meditation and the I Ching

Bruce Frantzis

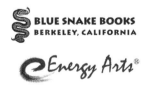

BLUE SNAKE BOOKS
BERKELEY, CALIFORNIA

Energy Arts®

Published by Blue Snake Books, an imprint of North Atlantic Books
P.O. Box 12327, Berkeley, California 94712
and
Energy Arts, Inc. Publications
P. O. Box 99, Fairfax, California 94978

The following trademarks are used under license by Energy Arts, Inc., from Bruce Frantzis: Frantzis Energy Arts® system, Mastery Without Mystery®, Longevity Breathing® program, Opening the Energy Gates of Your Body™ Qigong, Marriage of Heaven and Earth™ Qigong, Bend the Bow™ Spinal Qigong, Spiraling Energy Body™ Qigong, Gods Playing in the Clouds™ Qigong, Living Taoism™ Collection, Chi Rev Workout™, *Energy Arts*® and HeartChi®.

North Atlantic Books is part of the Society for the Study of Native Arts and Sciences, a nonprofit educational corporation whose goals are to develop an educational and cross-cultural perspective linking various scientific, social and artistic fields; to nurture a holistic view of arts, sciences, humanities and healing; and to publish and distribute literature on the relationship of mind, body and nature.

Cover design: Thomas Herington, Energy Arts, Inc.
Cover art: Abra Brayman
Interior design: Lisa Petty, GirlVibe, Inc.
Illustrations: Michael McKee
Cover Photo: Caroline Frantzis
Back Cover Photos: Richard Marks, Caroline Frantzis

Printed in the United States of America

PLEASE NOTE: The practice of Taoist energy arts, martial arts and the meditative arts may carry risks. The information in this book is not in any way intended as a substitute for medical, psychological or emotional counseling with a licensed physician or healthcare provider. The reader should consult a professional before undertaking any martial arts, movement, meditation, health or exercise program to reduce the chance of injury or any other harm that may result from pursuing or trying any technique discussed in this book. Any physical or other distress experienced during or after any exercise should not be ignored and should be brought to the attention of a healthcare professional. The creators and publishers of this book disclaim any liabilities for loss in connection with following any of the practices described in this book, and implementation is at the discretion, decision and risk of the reader.

Library of Congress Cataloging-in-Publication Data

Frantzis, Bruce Kumar.
 Bagua and Tai Chi : exploring the potential of Chi, martial arts,
meditation, and the I Ching / by Bruce Frantzis.
   p. cm.
 Includes bibliographical references.
 ISBN 978-1-58394-359-5 (pbk.)
 1. Tai chi--Health aspects. 2. Martial arts--Health aspects. I. Title.
 RA781.F677 2012
 613.7'046--dc23
                2011029093

1 2 3 4 5 6 7 8 9 Peter Schultz Printing 17 16 15 14 13 12

I dedicate this book to my main teacher,
Taoist Lineage Master Liu Hung Chieh of Beijing, China,
without whose generosity it could never have been written.

CONTENTS

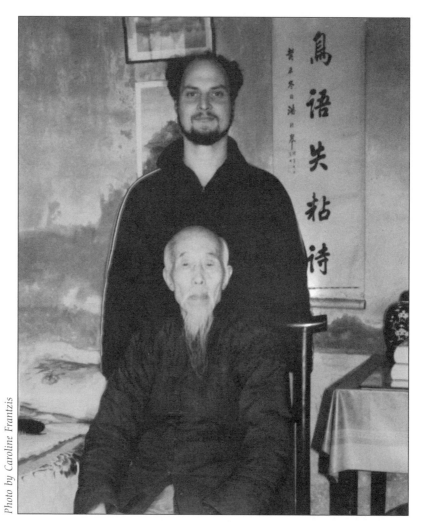

Taoist Lineage Master, Liu Hung Chieh, with his disciple, Bruce Frantzis. This photograph was taken in 1986 in Liu's home in Beijing, China.

ACKNOWLEDGMENTS

Many people graciously gave their time and effort during the development of this book. Special appreciation goes to three people: Bill Ryan, Senior Energy Arts Instructor and founder of Brookline Tai Chi and Toward Harmony Tai Chi and Qigong, for editorial and technical assistance; Heather Hale for editing and personal assistance; and my wife Caroline for editing, photographs and her never-ending inspiration and support.

I would also like to thank Diane Rapaport for developmental editing; Thomas Herington, Energy Arts, Inc. Administrative Assistant, for cover design; Lisa Petty, GirlVibe, Inc., for interior design and production; Richard Marks, Eric Peters, Mark Thayer and Bill Walters for photography; Nancy Riccio for organizational editing; Mountain Livingston, Energy Arts, Inc. Office Manager, for graphics and image coordination; Michael McKee for illustrations; and Kaualani Pereira and Energy Arts Instructors Bill Ryan, Paul Cavel, Craig Barnes and Lee Burkins for modeling movements.

I'm also grateful to the following people for their feedback and advice: Rich Taubinger, Stuart Kenter, Paul Cavel, Isaac Kamins and Jess O'Brien.

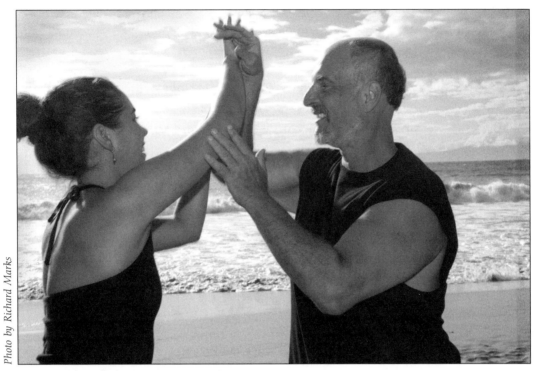

Photo by Richard Marks

The author teaches Tai Chi Push Hands. The first stage in Push Hands is to be able to center and root your energy, and reach a level where your opponent's energy and power never touch you. It's an art of playing with your own energy and that of your partner, and of building internal power.

INTRODUCTION

The aim of this book is to help you bring Taoism to life within your being. Although the great Taoist philosophical and spiritual books—including the *I Ching (Book of Changes)*, the *Tao Te Ching* by Lao Tse and the *Book of Chuang Tse*—are well known and available in many translations, the practical methods and techniques of implementing Taoist concepts in daily life are little known in the West. The manner in which they take root and flower is by strengthening chi (qi) flow in your mind, body and spirit. These practices have been in continual use in China for more than 4,000 years.

This book takes two of Taoism's greatest chi movement practices—bagua zhang and tai chi chuan—and describes what is required to progressively, concretely and pragmatically develop and embody high levels of chi flow. Optimizing your chi has potential multifaceted benefits. It can improve your overall health as well as help you become, for example, a highly productive entrepreneur, accomplished athlete, skilled martial artist or effective healer.

Working with chi can also take you far beyond your normal daily life, allowing you to embark on a profound spiritual path.

A Fusion of Exercise, Chi and Meditation

During my education in various modes of healing, martial arts and spirituality in America, Japan, India and China, I found no other systems that so seamlessly fused exercise and meditation into one integrated mind/body/spirit practice as bagua and tai chi.

When you begin to learn these arts, you quickly understand that they are primarily sophisticated, low-impact exercises that enable you to physically embody the principles of Chinese medicine and qigong. They systematically and progressively cultivate vibrant health and well-being from deep inside your being.

As you learn and practice, you recognize the movement of chi in your body on increasingly subtle levels. Aspects of internal power help you develop chi. Simultaneously, you use the movements as sophisticated tension-relief exercises that release and mitigate the corrosive acid of stress that eats away at your body—and your quality of life in general. Practitioners find that the more stress they release, the healthier they become. Who couldn't do with less stress and better health? Stress is the most prevalent disease of our modern age.

Not only can bagua and tai chi make you incredibly healthy and relaxed, but also these arts can build the foundation for meditation. You train your mind how to be relaxed, calm and focused. Very few modern exercise systems can boast this benefit, and many create physical strain. This may make the mind incredibly tense during practice, causing the opposite of relaxation.

These are some of the reasons why practitioners of the internal martial arts keep practicing throughout their lifetimes. Like any exercise system, you go from plateau to plateau, but there is no ultimate goal. You can continue developing your practice well into old age because your practice evolves as you do.

Pain, negative emotions and stress can sap your life force and distract you from reaching your potential. As you become healthier you increase your productivity and feel more youthful and alive.

Maintaining health and relaxation is the motivation for 99 percent of all people who practice bagua or tai chi. In fact, the majority of people in China, and many in the West, learn tai chi after the age of fifty, when the limitations of aging and beginnings of chronic disease commonly begin to surface.

Taoism: A Living Tradition

Taoism is a living tradition because chi development practices are not taught purely as intellectual or philosophical precepts. Physical practice, including the powerful exercises of bagua and tai chi (and other arts such as qigong, qigong tui na and hsing-i), help you realize the teachings. These exercises can make you exceptionally healthy, strong and relaxed. As you progress, you can work toward fulfilling your spiritual potential—should you so choose. Bagua and tai chi provide the exercise that your body needs to function well, while simultaneously developing your meditation skills. These include the basics, such as making the mind calmer and more focused, as well as more profound skills, such as finding stillness deep within your being.

The art and science of developing chi in the internal martial arts, including bagua and tai chi, is done by using the sixteen neigong components of internal power (discussed in detail in Chapter 2). Incorporating each of these elements separately, layer by layer, into your movements improves the quality and depth of your practice.

This ancient and pragmatic neigong system for tapping into chi was the main focus of my training in China. Practicing these arts gave me a structure that allowed chi to emerge and flourish within me. It can do the same for you.

Forms of Moving Meditation

Bagua and tai chi, when practiced as Taoist meditation, can eventually go beyond achieving the goals of relieving stress and calming the mind, and give you access to the highest spiritual potential—entering the realm of the sublime. As you progress on your spiritual journey, you use the movement practices of bagua and tai chi together with Taoist meditation to increasingly free your soul from deeper psychic and karmic aspects that bind you. You tap into the chi that connects you and the whole of the universe, known as the *Tao* or "universal consciousness."

Complete spiritual awakening is possible.

This book explains how the methods of bagua and tai chi can lead you on a profound spiritual journey that embodies the tenets and meditation practices of the Taoist tradition. These methods are not often accessible to Western students because few teachers are available who know the practices and are willing to teach them.

I was fortunate to learn the Taoist Water tradition within bagua and tai chi from Lineage Master Liu Hung Chieh. The lineage of masters to which I belong comes directly from and goes back to Lao Tse, author of the *Tao Te Ching,* who lived in antiquity.

The spiritual practices of bagua and tai chi make chi a living, felt force inside you at the very core of your spirit. In China, they say philosophers are like good scholars who know all the words, but practitioners embody the words and their meanings.

Value for All Aspects of Life

Bagua and Tai Chi has been written from the perspective of a Taoist Lineage Holder, one whose responsibility is to do his best to ensure that the chi-development arts of Taoism survive without degeneration. This is not just for the current or next generation, but for many generations beyond ours. The goal is to present an in-depth look at how the living reality of chi can be embedded in a person through two of the spirit and energy practices that underpin Taoism's meditation and somatic healing therapies.

This book was conceived to enable those not intimately familiar with Taoism to gain insight into how it approaches spirituality through the means of thoroughly engaging in the Taoist movement practices of bagua and tai chi. It will demonstrate how exercise can go beyond the ordinary and become exceptionally sophisticated.

Even if you were never to personally engage in these practices beyond their value for health and relaxation, you might get some ideas of ways to approach the subtleties of mind and spirit. Perhaps reading this text may yield some valuable insights into your own life path and forms of meditation to further your spiritual journey.

My goal is to present readers with a coherent idea of what it means to embody energy and meditation practices. I'm not interested in presenting abstract, intellectual theories. I want to give you a taste of the living reality of chi in the context of its immense value for life and its ability to instill internal peace, stability, joy, compassion and balance in your life.

The practices of bagua and tai chi are likened to seeds that are planted inside you. Once there, they grow and help transform you, often in the most surprisingly, unpredictable and wonderful ways, providing an endless source of creativity. As your practice nurtures these seeds, they grow into a tree that year after year bears more life-sustaining fruit.

My hope is that each succeeding generation can use these practices. With them, we gain the realistic possibility of working toward physical well-being, abundant life-force energy, peace of mind and an awakened spirit.

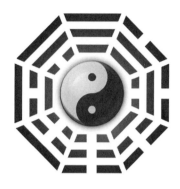

CHAPTER 1
An Overview of Bagua and Tai Chi

Two of China's great gifts to the world are the movement arts of bagua and tai chi. Although tai chi is far better known throughout the contemporary world, bagua is far older and some would say richer. It was developed more than 4,000 years ago as a Taoist health exercise and meditation art. During the past two centuries, however, bagua has become better known as a martial art called *bagua zhang* or "Eight Trigrams Palm Boxing."

Tai chi was developed several hundred years ago as a martial art. During the past century, however, it has become increasingly practiced for its potent health benefits and to develop such foundations for meditation as relaxation and calmness of mind. Tai chi can be used as a practical bridge toward the more profound aspects of Taoist meditation.

Bagua and tai chi share many similarities. Both practices are rooted in Taoism, a Chinese philosophical and spiritual tradition, and are designed to help develop and balance one's chi or life-force energy. They are expressions through the physical body of such Taoist concepts as yin-yang, balance and naturalness.

Although bagua and tai chi have important differences, they are wonderfully complementary brother and sister practices.

Tai chi is known as the sister because in its initial learning stages it strategically approaches the great art of chi more from a yin-energy approach. Bagua is the brother because its beginning practices approach chi more from a yang-energy approach.

Both arts include each other's yin and yang strengths and special qualities with only slight areas of differentiation. They equally share the ability to access and develop important and innate potential human abilities.

Arts of Movement and Chi Development

Bagua and tai chi can develop the art of movement to very sophisticated degrees, particularly through their methods for developing the chi of the body, mind and spirit.

Tai Chi

All forms of tai chi are performed as a sequence of flowing movements. Each carries your body into a particular posture from which you then move in a flowing manner to the next one. Your arms and legs move simultaneously in various directions: up and down, forward and back, right and left, outward and inward.

Almost all tai chi forms that most people learn today are done in slow motion and in very specific ways that are designed to relax the body and release nervous tension. A primary goal is to help your body and mind become comfortable as you get all the exercise that you need for health and wellness.

Tai chi short forms are typically comprised of about twenty movements; long forms usually include more than one hundred movements; and medium-length forms are somewhere in between. In longer tai chi forms, specific circular movement patterns continuously repeat several times throughout the entire set of movements.

Bagua

In bagua, you learn precise footwork methods for walking in circles in opposite directions. During early stages of learning, your hands are kept at your sides. Eventually, you learn to hold your hands in various postures, which are similar to, but not the same as, some of the postures used in tai chi.

As your training progresses you learn increasingly complex ways of changing direction, which includes footwork and hand movements. The various combinations of arm movements, used with the stepping actions of the legs as you reverse direction, are called *palm changes.* The most important and foundational palm change is the Single Palm Change.

Walking the Circle, as it is called in bagua, is customarily done at about the speed you might use when you walk down the street. In time, walking gets progressively faster until you speed walk. At this point, bagua becomes aerobic—a characteristic that distinguishes it from almost all forms of tai chi.

Unlike tai chi, bagua is not normally done in slow motion. Bagua is practiced in slow motion for short periods of time to develop physical coordination or balance. After the skill is grasped, you then go back to practicing at normal or fast speeds.

Chi Development

All forms of bagua and tai chi are designed to increase and balance your chi. You may choose to apply your chi in five primary areas:
- Health and/or high performance
- Longevity and regeneration
- Martial arts
- Healing
- Meditation

Health and High Performance

Bagua and tai chi can maximize your physical and mental health in the short and medium term (five to twenty years), while increasing your overall level of mental and physical vitality, strength and stamina. In the modern age this is usually enough for most people.

Developing truly superior physical, mental and spiritual functions is more challenging. This includes learning how to embody neigong components in dramatically greater depth in your movements. Neigong is the art and science of developing chi, which has its roots in the *I Ching.*

A drive toward high performance is commonly associated with type A personalities, who also unfortunately have a tendency toward excessive behaviors and over-straining the body. In this regard, a critical part of the training is learning to avoid injuries and the burnout that sadly often accompanies the attempt to acquire high-performance capabilities (see pp. 84–86 on the 70 percent rule).

Longevity and Regeneration

Living well into your old age, so that your golden years are truly enjoyed, provides strong motivation for learning bagua and tai chi. These practices help prevent disease and injury and—should stress and illness occur—enable you to recover and heal more quickly. They are rejuvenation tools. These important goals apply equally to youngsters who look forward to living many years, or people in their fifties and sixties who may suffer from stress and chronic disease.

Many who learn bagua and tai chi, even those that begin in their forties or fifties, find they become as capable mentally, physically and sexually as they were in their twenties and thirties. That is why these practices are considered keys to the real elixir of youth.[1]

Many bagua and tai chi practitioners believe that these arts may extend your actual years on the earth, although this is impossible to quantify. Factors beyond poor health can cause life to end suddenly. Nevertheless, many bagua and tai chi practitioners function at superlative levels of human physical and mental capacity until the day they die.

Martial Arts

Bagua and tai chi serve as training for attaining high levels of internal power, which can make you an effective fighter. These arts give you the ability to instantaneously, efficiently and upon demand release internal power to achieve your goals with maximum speed and coordination. Ideally, you learn to do this without damaging your body or mind and while maintaining optimum health.

There is always a potential price to pay at all levels of your being. These include testing your martial capabilities through physical combat, including physical pain, or potential injury from contests and competitions or using martial skills in real-life war or law-enforcement situations.

---

[1] See Appendix A, which discusses the applications and benefits of bagua and tai chi at all stages of life.

Likewise, part of the cost is the unstinting effort you must sustain to learn, test and prove yourself as you achieve progressively more difficult and challenging degrees of skill.

Healing

If your goal is to heal others—physically, emotionally, mentally or psychically—bagua and tai chi can help you develop the chi you will need.

First, these practices will increase your personal energy. In the process you can learn how to channel and use energy from the external environment, outside your body, so you can transmit it to others. The techniques will help you develop your intuition and a type of somatic intelligence that enhances your healing abilities. This process also enables you to become sensitive to the energies of others and develop compassion as you work with your patients.

Bagua and tai chi will help you acquire energetic skills so that you can stay healthy and unstressed. Preventing burnout is a primary application. As any healthcare professional or bodyworker knows, protecting yourself from the chi of your patients or clients is critical to maintaining your vitality and being able to continue your healing career for the long haul.

Meditation

When practiced as meditation, bagua and tai chi are unique in that they seamlessly fuse exercise and meditation. They give you practical methods to become healthier while providing profound spiritual practices. You can engage in exercise and meditation simultaneously rather than doing one at a time.

If at some point you have the opportunity to practice bagua and tai chi within a genuine Taoist meditation tradition, then you will go beyond movements that help you get healthier and calm your mind. You will engage in a profound spiritual path, which can enable you to become emotionally and mentally balanced and mature, as well as take you to the deeper, mental, emotional, psychic and karmic aspects of your being.

At this level, meditation helps you become fully conscious of the chi of your physical body. Later, you can deal with the deeper matters of your spirit and essence, which is usually unconscious and/or trapped in the body. If you manage to release your blockages at these levels, then you will become fully awake at all levels of human consciousness.

THE EXERCISE-MEDITATION CONTINUUM

When you practice bagua or tai chi as Taoist meditation, at no point is there a distinct dividing line between when you are exercising and when you are meditating. They become two sides of the same coin. By shining and refining the coin from both sides at once, you progressively open your heart to receiving two gifts for the price of one: exquisite exercise and profound spiritual realization.

Refining the exercise side of the coin helps your bagua or tai chi progress from a beginning qigong exercise toward becoming an ever more finely tuned movement art. The root becomes the sixteen neigong components through which your body can handle the increasingly powerful energies inside and outside you that release in meditation.

Shining the meditation side of the coin initially helps you gain heightened levels of awareness. Together with emotional and mental stability and clarity, it turns you toward exploration of the most refined and profound spiritual energies within your inner and outer worlds.

In order to support spiritual exploration, your body and mind must become progressively more healthy, open and alive. It is the only way that the more powerful energies of the universe can smoothly—rather than disjointedly—move through you. It is only when these energies are available to you that you can fully make your body and mind healthy, open and alive.

Of course old age, illness or injury can catch up with everyone, so the inherent limitations of the body will sooner or later prevail. However, for most bagua and tai chi practitioners this potential pain and discomfort is typically significantly mitigated. Even so, the farther along the Taoist exercise-meditation continuum one travels, the more capacity you will have to more smoothly manage and navigate the limitations of your physical body. With it, you will experience the balance, joy and inner freedom that meditation brings.

If you take bagua or tai chi to their most profound levels, your spirit may become capable of extending beyond your body to connect and join with the Tao, or universal consciousness.

Taoist Meditation Arts of the *I Ching*

Thousands of years ago the art of bagua was developed by Taoist monks as a form of moving meditation based on the principles of the *I Ching (Book of Changes)*. Some of its principles include the interplay of change between yin and yang, and the transcendence of yin and yang that leads to what is eternal, permanent and unchanging. It is known by such names as the Tao, primordial space, emptiness and the universal link that connects all and everything.

Complete study of the *I Ching* includes advanced practices in bagua. Here you can literally coordinate all levels of your being—physical, energetic, emotional, mental, psychic, karmic and spiritual—with the five primal energies (also known as the Five Elements) of manifestation.

My teacher Liu taught me how to adapt the principles of the *I Ching* into Wu style tai chi, a process that Liu learned with Taoist elders during ten years of training in the mountains of Sichuan Province in the 1940s.

Bagua and tai chi broaden the possibilities of movement arts beyond their martial and health traditions into the realms of meditation. Practice will help you:

- Accept and flow with change.
- Understand the spiritual quality of emptiness.
- Become one with the ever-changing universe, your own unchanging consciousness and ultimately with universal consciousness, or the Tao.

Similar pathways can also be pursued through tai chi, although tai chi forms were not originally developed specifically for purposes of Taoist meditation. It was adapted for this purpose in the twentieth century as tai chi grew in popularity. With a focus on the interplay of yin and yang, tai chi forms can be well-suited as vessels for embodying the principles of the *I Ching*.

Heart-Mind: The Center of Your Awareness

From the perspective of Taoist meditation, bagua and tai chi are arts of awareness above all else.

Meditation practices eventually lead to two interesting questions: Where is the origin of thought? Where is the origin of awareness itself? With enough practice, you move into what the Chinese call *hsin,* or the "Heart-Mind," which is on the edge of internal alchemy or energy transformation. You are not fully immersed in alchemy yet, but moving in that direction.

At this level of meditation, you work with the techniques of the Heart-Mind, which allow your awareness to perceive the place where thoughts originate. You discover what a thought actually is while becoming acutely aware of the consciousness that generates it in the first place. A deep awareness enables you to recognize and interpret it.

Most of us right now can recognize the existence of thought, a conversation in your head—whether scientific, intellectual, philosophical or something mundane. Maybe you're thinking about what you ate for breakfast. Ordinary thinking represents a certain type of mental activity that virtually everyone will acknowledge is present.

But when you go to the place from which the consciousness that literally travels from birth to death is generated, you reach a middle ground. In meditation, this is the point from which you deal with consciousness. In Lao Tse's Water method of meditation, you use dissolving techniques to go through the mind flow, next the emotions, eventually discovering the place from which thought is produced. You literally follow the mindstream to the edge of the direct experience of consciousness itself.

When your conscious awareness arrives at this destination, you can use all sorts of techniques to unravel the knots in your consciousness to completely free your spirit.

BAGUA MASTERY PROGRAM™ OVERVIEW

The Bagua Mastery Program is the most comprehensive bagua training program ever developed for the internal martial arts. You can use it to learn and practice bagua by itself or with the help of a bagua teacher. Learn more and sign up for more information here: www.energyarts.com/bagua-zhang-training.

Message from Bruce

When I initially left New York in the 1970s to study martial arts in the Far East, I was considered an outsider. To gain access I knew that I would be required to do at least two things. First of all I had to learn the relevant languages. Thus I practiced and became fluent in both Japanese and Chinese. Learning the native languages was the only way that I would be able to truly understand the teachings.

The second requirement was to show up and practice longer and with more intensity than everyone around me because that was the only way the masters would teach a foreigner. During this time I lived and breathed martial arts 24/7. I was put to the test mentally, emotionally, physically and eventually spiritually. I persevered through many challenges and hardships.

Because I learned the languages and practiced with discipline, many of the teachers took me under their wing. They saw that I would both practice what they taught me and help keep the real arts alive by teaching them to others. There was an implicit assumption that I would help carry the teachings forward or, at the very least, practice the arts to the highest possible level.

The real opportunity for every practitioner is to first realize the immense power of tai chi and bagua. These arts literally transform your life. They can be practiced for martial arts, improving your health, becoming a better healer, and especially for meditation and spiritual growth.

In the world today you can buy information on any subject; however, this is very different from actually extracting the value from that information. This can only be done through practice. When you follow precise methods and work with an initiated teacher you get results. These are results that you embody. Then your knowledge becomes a living reality. You gain an internal treasure.

I know that when I practiced bagua for the first time, I realized something very different was happening to the energetics of my body. Walking in a circle is very powerful especially with specific hand postures or palm changes. Doing so activates everything in your body, especially your major energetic channels. Bagua lets you manifest the energies of the *I Ching* within your eight energy bodies.

The way I learned bagua was unique because I was taught both the martial arts tradition of bagua and the monastic tradition which uses bagua for meditation and spiritual growth, something that to my knowledge is unique even in China. I wanted to pass on this knowledge to the next generation. Thus the Bagua Mastery Program was born.

The Bagua Mastery Program is a comprehensive program to teach you bagua. The program is also extremely beneficial if you practice tai chi because all the internal components of bagua are utilized in tai chi as well. We offer this program only periodically. Please read further to find out more about the program.

Be well,

Bruce Frantzis
Founder, Energy Arts

BAGUA MASTERY PROGRAM HIGHLIGHTS

The Bagua Mastery Program contains twelve modules. During the program you receive:

- Over 1,000 pages of step-by-step training materials
- Guided practice sessions on 16 audio CDs
- 35 DVDs taken from our live Bagua Instructor Training, Bagua Wind Palm and Bagua Earth Palm events
- An exclusive membership to an online community of bagua practitioners with access to forums, videos, audio files and other special bonuses

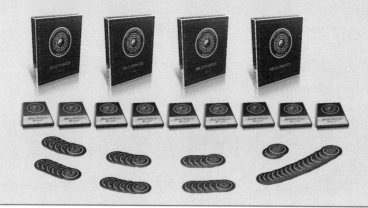

BAGUA MASTERY MODULES

The Bagua Mastery Program is composed of twelve consecutive training modules. Traditionally, bagua would be taught to dedicated students over a period of three to ten years. This material is presented in a way that you can learn at your own pace according to your ability.

Module 1 - Bagua Foundation Building: In this module you will build the historical context for learning bagua. You will learn the Bagua Internal Warm-up Method™ and be introduced to the Bagua Dynamic Stepping System™, the foundation for bagua walking techniques.

Module 2 - Bagua Circle Walking: Circle Walking can give your body all the aerobic exercise it needs. It brings up a vortex of energy from the earth through your body, which energizes, nourishes and strengthens your body from the inside out. It also sets the stage for using Circle Walking in Taoist meditation.

Module 3 - Bagua Body Unification and Direction Changes: The simplified turn for changing direction while Walking the Circle will be taught in this module. It works out the basic mechanics of getting used to reversing direction—including maintaining your balance and not getting disoriented. You will also learn the Bagua Body Unification Method™ in this module, which is comprised of three powerful exercises that unify your body.

Module 4 - Bagua Energy Postures: In Module 4, the circle of learning begins anew. You will learn my Bagua Energy Posture Series. A bagua energy posture involves the position of your arms being fixed in relation to your body while you Walk the Circle. Bagua energy postures, like the standing postures of tai chi, hsing-i and qigong, are used to develop a strong foundation for all moving practices in the world of chi.

Module 5 - Bagua Single Palm Change Posture: Holding the palm posture of the Single Palm Change (SPC) while Walking the Circle focuses and develops the chi of the body, mind and spirit more than any other independent single technique in the world of Taoist chi arts. It has tremendous value on every level, from health to spirituality.

Module 6 - Bagua Dragon Body: The Dragon Body is distinct to bagua. It should only be learned after stabilizing the Single Palm Change posture. The Dragon Body's form has the following two qualities as you Walk the Circle: the waist turns toward the center of the circle, and the torso maintains the four points and all of the other alignments of the preceding sections.

Module 7 - Bagua Complete Direction Change and Advanced Energy Postures: You will learn the complete footwork for changing and reversing the circle's direction. First, you use a toe-in step to turn your torso from the waist and shrink your body into itself, toward your body's centerline. Then, you use a toe-out step to turn your torso to the outside of your body's centerline and in the opposite direction from which you started.

Module 8 - Bagua Single Palm Change Warm-up: In this module, you will learn a physical and energetic warm-up that will help make the Single Palm Change one single, fluid movement as you change directions while Walking the Circle. The central goal of the Single Palm Change warm-up is to integrate arm movements with foot movements as you Walk the Circle. Later, because you'll be familiar enough with the movements already, changing direction won't be so overwhelming.

Module 9 - Bagua Heaven Single Palm Change and Changing Directions: All of the techniques and principles in the previous modules will now be applied as one integrated whole while you Walk the Circle and change direction using the Single Palm Change. This module puts all of the components you have learned together so you can do the Heaven Single Palm Change. Once you have reached this module, you'll have already built a solid foundation from which to learn the Single Palm Change.

Module 10 - Bagua Water Single Palm Change and Roll the Ball: The Water Single Palm Change trains you in the complexity of the spiraling arm actions. Although best learned through live instruction, learning to perform this palm change well has immense value.

Module 11 - Bagua Double Palm Change: The Bagua Double Palm Change is represented by the second trigram of the *I Ching*, known as "earth" (or *kun* in Chinese). It signifies the essence of yin energy as the prime yin or soft power generation method of bagua. This module teaches all of the components of this palm change.

Module 12 - Bagua Wind Palm Change: The Wind Palm Change develops the spinning techniques of bagua whereby the practitioner's body spins like a whirlwind. This module teaches all of the components of this palm change.

LEARN MORE

To find out more about the Bagua Mastery Program please visit the following website and join our list to find out the next time it will be released: *www.energyarts.com/bagua-zhang-training*.

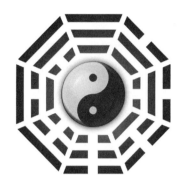

CHAPTER 2
Qigong and Neigong in Bagua and Tai Chi

How I Learned Taoist Chi Practices

My interest in the martial, healing and meditation arts started in my youth in Manhattan and flowered during my teens. At the age of eighteen, I went to Japan for intensive study and had the good fortune to discover Morehei Ueshiba, the founder of aikido. I was introduced in depth to the power of chi or life-force energy.

However, it was only after I went to Taiwan and met Wang Shu Jin, the great Chinese bagua master, that I began to fully pursue the Taoist path of warrior/healer/priest. I became fluent in Mandarin Chinese, lived in Taiwan and Hong Kong for seven years and studied martial arts intensively with many of its renowned masters. I also worked as a qigong tui na healer (energy bodyworker) in Chinese medical clinics and became a Taoist priest.

In 1981, through unusual circumstances, I was accepted as a formal disciple of the eminent Taoist Lineage Holder Liu Hung Chieh in Beijing. Although one of my masters had given me a letter of introduction to Liu, the main reason he accepted me was that he had a prophetic dream about teaching Taoist practices to a foreigner. It was one of only a few dreams Liu had had in his entire life, all of which came to pass.

After many initial conversations and training, my teacher Liu asked me a question: "Since you know at least some of the rudiments of qigong, have a little skill as a martial artist and served as a qigong tui na doctor, would you like to learn the essential core of Taoist chi practices, including its spiritual traditions?"

I most gratefully said yes.

Some years later when Liu said I had understood these core principles, he passed on his lineages in the Taoist Water tradition to me.[1] To this day, I consider myself incredibly fortunate to have learned the complete traditions of bagua zhang, tai chi chuan, Taoist qigong and Taoist meditation from him. These are truly the greatest treasures that the universe allowed me to bring from China.[2]

The Water Method of Taoism

Within Taoism, as with all spiritual traditions, are various schools of practice and thought. My teacher Liu specifically trained me in the Taoist Water tradition, which is closely allied with the ancient teaching of Lao Tse and Chuang Tse and includes the sixteen-part neigong system. The other branch is known as the Fire tradition, surfacing approximately 1,000 years ago in such schools as the Clear Reality School of Taoism.

What Is a Lineage Master?

In China, Taoist energy arts have been passed down through hundreds of generations by lineage holders. As with any discipline, there is a ladder or hierarchy of learning, comparable to the process a student undergoes starting at elementary school to learn the basics of a given subject and ending up with a PhD and chair at a major university.

Practitioners of internal energy arts (qigong, bagua, tai chi and hsing-i) include beginning, junior and senior students; as well as masters, disciples and lineage

---

[1] See Appendix D for specific details of these lineages.
[2] See Epilogue for conversations the author had with his teacher Liu about the best ways to progressively and effectively introduce chi practices to the West.

masters. Senior students usually take classes with a master; masters can become the formal disciples of lineage holders. Lineage holders are specifically trained by the lineage holder that preceded them. Only a lineage holder can pass down the lineage.

A lineage holder knows the whole of a Taoist tradition, not just its discrete parts, from its martial arts and health aspects to meditation. That person would know the complete sixteen-part neigong system and how each component is applied at various stages of practice and for what purposes (such as health, healing, martial arts or spirituality). The lineage holder would understand the major Taoist philosophical and spiritual texts and how they integrate into the chi arts and Taoist meditation.

Historically, the higher level chi arts were taught one-on-one or in small groups after disciples had trained and prepared sufficiently to absorb and embody the knowledge relatively smoothly. This is partially because, at the advanced levels of learning, disciples and lineage holders teach these practices and impart their knowledge by direct transmission of energy.

Functionally, about 4,000 to 5,000 channels of energy run through a human being. The only way to understand how to feel and use them—whether for health, healing, martial arts, high performance or spirituality—is to have someone directly transmit them to you over long periods of training so that you are unambiguous about what you feel. This is why live training is so important.

Then, you practice the applications on your own or in relation to others. For example, I used healing techniques of qigong, Wu style tai chi and Taoist meditation to completely heal my back from a horrendous car accident that resulted in several cracked vertebrae. In the decade that I studied and worked in China as a qigong healer, I treated thousands of people who had bone damage, organ problems and nerve disorders, including spending more than a year treating many patients with advanced cancer.

The necessity of learning from direct transmissions is the reason Chinese masters are so concerned with lineages: what exactly was taught, who studied with whom, where they got their knowledge and how the system was developed or conceived in the first place.

The Path of Liu Hung Chieh

In his early conversations with me, my teacher Liu described his own path of learning the Taoist energy arts. He too had followed the path of warrior/healer/priest from youth. He began studying martial arts at the age of eleven and, by the age of thirty, was a grandmaster of bagua and head of the instructors at the Hunan Branch of the Central Government's National Martial Arts Association. Two of his junior instructors were Wu Jien Chuan's sons who taught him Wu style tai chi. Later, Liu became Wu Jien Chuan's formal disciple and lived in Master Wu's house in Hong Kong, where he learned the deepest levels of the Wu style.

Liu added that although he had learned parts of the medical implications of bagua as a youth (family members had been Chinese doctors for ten generations), it was only after he spent a decade in the Southwest China province of Sichuan, before returning to Beijing in Northern China, that he finished learning the complete Taoist medical qigong, martial art and spiritual tradition of the sixteen-part neigong system. During this time, Liu also became one of the rare few to head a lineage of a small, but very important ancient Taoist sect. This lineage had directly passed down the teachings of Lao Tse in their purest forms to Liu's generation.

Liu also ascended and gained the right to be called a *Taoist Immortal* or what in Buddhism is often called a *Living Buddha.* With the rise of Communism in China, Liu returned to Beijing. There he lived out the rest of his life quietly, teaching only a few students and perfecting his own practice. The literary Chinese name Liu has given me as a lineage holder is Fan Qingren (Fan Zhishan is the spoken form of this name).

Chi and the Sixteen-Part Neigong System

The sixteen neigong components are energetic methods that in aggregate comprise all the specific subtle chi methodologies contained in each and every energy practice in China. These methods originally came from Taoist practices that will be discussed in detail in Chapter 3.

This system of energy work lies at the heart of bagua and tai chi as a means for developing chi. Each of the individual sixteen components has potentially hundreds of specific techniques and applications.

These are the components:[3]
1. Breathing methods, from the simple to progressively more complex
2. Feeling, moving, transforming and transmuting internal energies along the descending, ascending and connecting energy channels of the body
3. Precise external and internal body alignments to prevent the flow of chi from being blocked or dissipated
4. Dissolving physical, emotional and spiritual blockages
5. Moving energy through the main and secondary meridian channels of the body, including the energy gates
6. Lengthening, bending and stretching the body from the inside out and from the outside in along the direction of the yin and yang acupuncture meridian lines
7. Opening and closing all parts of the body's tissues (joints, muscles, soft tissues, internal organs, glands, blood vessels, cerebrospinal system and brain), as well as all the body's subtle energy anatomy from the outside in, along the direction of the yin and yang acupuncture meridian lines
8. Manipulating the energies and flows within the external aura outside the body
9. Making circles and spirals of energy inside the body, controlling the spiraling energy currents of the body and moving chi to any part of the body at will, especially to the glands, brain and internal organs
10. Absorbing energy into and projecting energy away from all parts of the body.
11. Controlling all the energies of the spine
12. Gaining control of the left and right energy channels of the body
13. Gaining control of the central energy channel of the body
14. Developing the capabilities and all the uses of the body's lower tantien
15. Developing the capabilities and all the uses of the body's upper and middle tantiens
16. Integrating all fifteen previous components and connecting every part of the physical body into one, unified energy

Even a quick scan through these neigong components reveals the sophistication required to teach bagua or tai chi as a complete, classic qigong practice. The best bagua and tai chi practitioners know some or most neigong elements, but only a rare few know and teach the complete system.

---

[3] The energy anatomy of the human body is shown in Appendix C.

QIGONG, BAGUA AND TAI CHI: SIMILARITIES AND DIFFERENCES

The Taoist movement practices of qigong, bagua and tai chi share fundamental principles of physical movement, development of internal energy flows and ways to direct the mind while practicing. All are based upon developing health and relaxation. Bagua and tai chi also have powerful methods that can lead you to develop the highest levels of Taoism's spiritual potential.

However, the strategies by which they accomplish their goals differ. Bagua has only one major movement (Circle Walking) and many ways of holding the hands (palm changes). Qigong has hundreds of styles and movement forms, and the composition of a specific form could range from a few physical movements to well over a hundred. There are five major styles of tai chi and, within each one, a form may have anywhere from sixteen to more than one hundred movements.

You could think of these practices as containers for the richness of the qualities they develop, comparable to how wine bottles hold a huge variety of wines. Their differences mostly apply to beginning practices of these arts. When they approach advanced levels, the differences tend to even out—if the system is complete.

The Taoist Concept of Chi

According to the Taoists, the universe is composed of energy, or chi. They believe that different types of energy combine to allow the 10,000 possibilities,[4] or all and everything that can manifest in the entire world.

In this way, Taoists were a few thousand years ahead of modern quantum theory that explores the interplay of the relationship between matter and energy. As their scientific explorations evolve, the theories of physicists seem to coincide with and verify the principles of energy that Taoists discovered millennia ago. Whereas modern physicists have uncovered the principles behind the mysteries of energy using mathematics and highly sophisticated forms of instrumentation, the sages of Taoism did so purely by having their awareness go incredibly deeply into their being.[5] They often sat alone in isolated places in nature.

---

4 "10,000" is actually a metaphor often used in Taoist texts to describe an infinite number of possibilities.
5 See *The Tao of Physics* by Fritjof Capra (Shambhala Publications, 2000) or *The Dancing Wu Li Masters* by Gary Zukav (HarperOne, 2001).

Taoists are very practical people who observe how nature repeats itself at macro and micro levels. They believe that if you could take any one manifestation or form of energy in this universe and understand it to its fullest depths, you could thereby understand all the energies of the entire universe. This is identical to taking any one small part of a hologram to recreate the whole hologram.

Embodying Chi

In the Taoist tradition, chi is a living reality inside you rather than just an idea or an aspiration. For example, you can imagine taking a drink all day, but until you actually take a sip you won't quench your thirst.

Taoist practices go beyond only thinking about philosophical and spiritual principles to embodying them. Chi becomes a live, felt force inside you. It literally becomes a part of your blood, bones and everything down to the absolute core of your soul.

The living qualities of chi can be felt as clearly and concretely inside you as when you hold something in your hand or bite your tongue. Chi development *begins* with movements that train you to feel chi at its quintessential physical level. In time and with practice, feeling and strengthening chi occurs on much more profound levels.

Chi powers both your positive and negative emotions and thoughts. How do you become aware and get rid of the chi of dysfunctional emotions or negative thought patterns that plague and imprison you? How do you become aware of the chi within you that has incredible spiritual content? How can you enable joy and compassion to flourish? Taoists have sought the answers to these questions for millennia to help people reach the pinnacle of health, martial ability and spirituality.[6]

Pragmatic Methods of Chi Development

Taoists developed numerous arts millennia ago, which are all concerned with developing chi in human beings. These arts include martial arts such as bagua and tai chi, fine arts such as painting and calligraphy, and Chinese medicine, which includes qigong, acupuncture, bone-setting and other health modalities. One of the highest levels of spiritual development—achieved through Taoist meditation—is to find the permanent, unchanging center of your being.

---

6 The applications of chi development in tai chi are discussed in depth in the author's book *Tai Chi: Health for Life*. The different ways chi is developed and applied in the martial arts of bagua, tai chi and hsing-i are found in his book *The Power of Internal Martial Arts and Chi*.

QIGONG'S CONNECTION WITH
BAGUA, TAI CHI AND TAOIST MEDITATION

Hundreds of years ago the term *qigong* was rarely used. Instead, the term *neigong*, derived from the sixteen-part neigong system, was more popular.

All Taoist meditation contains qigong. Conversely, qigong may not have anything to do with meditation. Qigong in Chinese means to "work with chi." Usually, qigong has to do with improving, strengthening and balancing the energy related to enhancing your physical and mental health. Practicing qigong within any standing, moving (such as bagua or tai chi) or sitting practice may only be for physical health or internal power generation. It may not have anything to do with meditation.

Meditation deals with the deepest qualities of the soul that go beyond purely biological needs. Meditation, at its deeper levels, revolves around issues that comprise the most powerful and subtle aspects of human stress, emotions, psychic sensitivities, karma and spiritual essence. Although bagua and tai chi are moving qigong forms that can make someone healthier, stronger and less stressed, they also include additional chi elements as genuine vehicles for meditation.

When ordinary qigong enters the world of meditation and spirituality, it becomes *shengong*, which literally translates as "spiritual qigong." Shengong deals with the qualities of chi that run a human being's higher energy bodies (see Chapter 3 on the eight energy bodies).

If bagua and tai chi are to become genuine forms of Taoist meditation, they must first be rooted in ordinary qigong. Once your practice is developed and stabilized, you seek to refine and clear the foundation—the first seven energy bodies—as a prelude to working with the core spiritual energies of the universe or the Tao.

Energy arts also include *feng shui* (literally "wind-water"), which is known in the West as geomancy. Feng shui is concerned with how the external energies of the earth, sun, sky, landscape and time affect human beings and the potential events connected to them. More pragmatically, feng shui is used to determine how to make the energy of all or part of a building harmonious with whom or what will inhabit that space. Still other chi arts involve the chi of politics, war, science, astrology and metaphysics.

All Taoist arts are essentially concerned with balancing and increasing chi. Taoists believe that if you could realize and embody these arts internally, they would eventually lead you to the primary meditation traditions of internal alchemy.

Internal alchemy is about:
- Freeing your spirit from the limitations of the human body
- Understanding how the universal forces work inside and outside you
- Changing your entire energy matrix
- Merging and become one with the universe

Different people have different natural interests and aptitudes. Taoists developed diverse internal arts to give people alternative frameworks or options through which profound spiritual essences could be realized. The skills needed to become a painter are different from those needed to be a doctor; those of a doctor are different from those needed by a martial artist; and those of a martial artist are different from those needed by a geomancer.

Taoists believed that it was best for an individual to initially become involved with whatever practices naturally resonated with their own particular interests. They advocated that this would further spiritual interests more than engaging in what people thought they *ought* to do.

Understanding how the flows of your own energies work and how to relax and follow them naturally removes unnecessary obstacles that can easily be avoided. It also provides insight into how energies universally manifest.

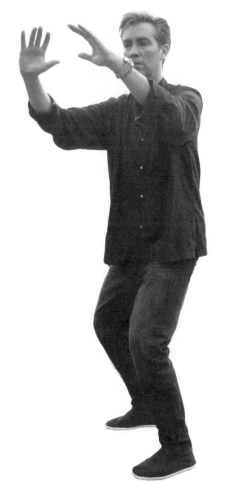

Photo courtesy of Craig Barnes

A posture from Gods Playing in the Clouds Qigong, an advanced set that integrates all sixteen neigong components and serves as a bridge to Taoist meditation.

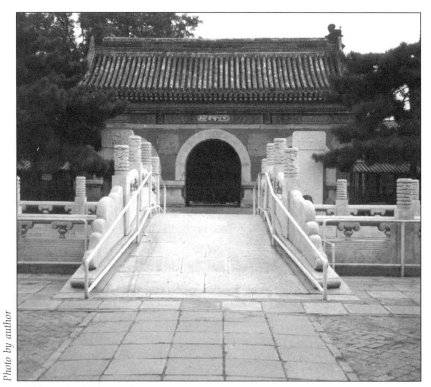

Photo by author

Gateway to the Inner Temple of the Bai Yun Guan (White Cloud Temple) in Beijing, China, one of the most important centers of Taoism in China. The author spent many hours here practicing the Taoist meditation methods that he learned from Lui Hung Chieh.

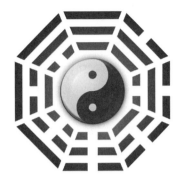

CHAPTER 3
What Is Taoism?

Taoism is one of the world's great living spiritual traditions, although in the West it has only recently come out of the shadows. According to oral tradition, Taoism came to China from the Kunlun Mountains, between northern Tibet and Central Asia's Takla Makan Desert, about 4,000 to 5,000 years ago.

The central spiritual teaching of Taoism is to restore balance in all aspects of our lives, including our physical bodies, daily affairs and relationships with others and the environment. Most importantly, Taoism teaches that through deep spiritual relaxation and balance we can reconnect directly to our innermost being. With this connection to our soul we can link with the source of the universe or the Tao.[1]

Taoism and China

Taoism began flourishing in China around the sixth century B.C. Yet it is little known and often confused with Buddhism.[2] Nonetheless, Taoism is alive and well today.

Taoism and Buddhism are unique spiritual expressions. As religions or spiritual paths, both have excellent and friendly relations with each other and share many

---

[1] The word *Tao* can also refer to the life path along which a person travels toward enlightenment.
[2] See Appendix B: "Why Buddhism and Hinduism Are Well Known, but Taoism Is Not."

common points. Yet neither comes from the other, each having very different historical roots.

Taoism was born before the Buddha lived, originated in China and hasn't yet spread much outside Asia. Buddhism arose and developed in India, then traveled and established itself widely all over the world. In China, Taoism and Buddhism began cross-fertilizing each other from about 1,000 to 1,500 years after Buddha's birth, although little cross-fertilization occurred in India. Buddhism is reported to be one of the fastest-growing religions in the modern world.

The bridge from China to the West is still under construction. Even when the British occupied China for some decades in the nineteenth century, few became fluent in Chinese. The language barrier has kept many of China's great books from being translated and its cultural and religious practices shrouded in mystery.

Moreover, most chi-development practices were quite secret, and few outsiders had easy access to learning them. I had to learn the language and prove myself to teachers in China time and again to gain access to advanced levels of practice.

Although the many faces of Taoism are new to us, they have existed in China for millennia.

China and Its Culture

Today, China is becoming a major world player. As Napoleon once commented about China, "I fear we have awakened the sleeping giant." Most public interest in and knowledge about China currently revolves around its politics and financial reserves, and whether China will be friend or foe in the future.

However, there is a completely different side of China, which from below the surface molds its thinking and actions, providing some insights into why historically it has become a giant that has risen many times before.

Taoism lies at the roots of Chinese culture and weaves through every facet of how the Chinese tend to think and act today. In many previous eras Taoism was at least as influential as Confucianism. Taoism forms a part of the underlying spiritual foundations of China's secular thought, just as Judaism and Christianity underlie Western culture in obvious and subtle ways. Today, Taoist thought frames how ordinary and sophisticated Chinese people think and influences their cultural conditionings.

ABOUT THE SPELLINGS OF CHINESE WORDS

Chinese has many sounds that do not exist in English or other European languages. All written Chinese words were not originally created from an alphabet. Most attempts by Westerns to render the basic sounds of the language into something that resembles what it actually sounds like in Chinese have been very vague approximations.

Currently, three standard transliteration systems attempt to render Chinese sounds into the written English alphabet. Generally, the Wade-Giles and Pinyin systems have poor representations of many primary Chinese sounds. Only the Yale system does a decent job of bridging the pronunciation gap with the English alphabet. Someone reading a Yale version, without knowing Chinese, might have a chance of getting somewhat close to what the term sounds like. This issue matters when attempting to communicate about the subjects with a native Chinese speaker who shares your interest.

For example, the full name of bagua in Chinese is rendered as "bagua zhang" in the Pinyin system, "pa kua chang" in the Wade-Giles system and "bagwa jang" in the Yale system. The translation of each into English is "eight trigram palm."

To make matters more complicated, a word like palm (and many others) is often not transliterated as it is even remotely pronounced in Chinese. For example, the sound of the first letter in the word for palm is closest to the "J" sound, but this is not quite so when it is combined with the "A" that follows it.

Before the 1970s, the Wade-Giles system was the most commonly used in academia. Today, the Pinyin system is the academic standard. Although the Yale system, which was created by Yale University in the early twentieth century, was specifically designed to make sense for Western audiences, it has never been widely used in popular books and magazines.

In this book, I have chosen to insert into the text whichever transliteration I believe will be of most use to the ordinary reader, rather than to the academic community. Therefore, this book uses either transliteration or spellings that are closest to their Chinese pronunciation and/or which, accurately or not, are the most commonly used in print.

Appendix E lists the various ways that the three transliteration systems spell Chinese terms and gives basic definitions.

My hope is to provide a window into how Taoist thought translates into real life. This includes when the Chinese make important decisions and pragmatically follow through on their ideas. By focusing very specifically on how bagua and tai chi shape the life force in the body, mind and spirit, this text can give you a sense of many aspects central to the Chinese cultural matrix—including the extreme importance placed on success through patience, follow-through and emphasis on the long term. Consistency is needed for effective implementation of every small phase over the long haul.

The Chinese study human subjects of health and spirituality in pursuit of what they think a refined or intelligent person would do to best serve their life's purpose while on this planet. The major principles of Taoism are found in its ancient texts, and eminent teachers have carried them forward within two of its greatest movement arts: bagua and tai chi.

These principles are also the basis of Traditional Chinese Medicine and meditation.

The Chinese approach goes above and beyond practical material issues like making money or pursuing power. Here, the philosophical underpinnings of the culture reveal themselves by the process of how complex skills are acquired.

The *I Ching*

The fundamental principles of Taoism originate from an intimate and thorough understanding of the *I Ching*. The *I Ching* is concerned with the underlying nature of energy and its manifestations of change within people and events throughout the universe.

The essential sections that comprise the *I Ching*, sometimes referred to as the "ancient texts," were written down more than 2,000 years ago. However, Taoists believe that these sections date back as far as 5,000 years and were developed by Taoist adepts who also passed down the essential sections through oral traditions for 8,000 years.

Although no one knows for sure, it seems that when these sections were written down, commentaries and interpretations were added. Experts differ in opinion about what is the original tradition and what is commentary or interpretation.

The *I Ching* is considered to be the bible of both the Fire and Water schools of Taoism. It is also the direct source of energetic principles that underlie bagua, tai chi and other Taoist energy arts. These include all the yin and yang principles, strategies for directing chi and mind flow patterns, and neigong—from the simple to complex.

Bagua and tai chi are methods through which you can bring to life and manifest the principles of the *I Ching* within your body, mind and spirit.

In both ancient and modern times, people have been using the *I Ching* as a tool of divination and mathematics, and as a book of wisdom. The *I Ching* mimics the underlying basis of computer code, which shows how relevant its applications are today.

Lao Tse and Chuang Tse

The great sages Lao Tse (circa sixth century B.C.) and Chuang Tse (circa fourth century B.C.) lived at a time when everything that comprises what we call life—sublime or of the gutter—was seen in the context of the sacred and mystical. They looked at life through the lens of what was useful. They constantly examined life's ordinary events in the context of emptiness and the Tao.

They did not purely focus on highly specific actions as determinants of morality, but rather on the spirit or awareness behind actions.

Both sages were opposite in character, but equally wise. Lao Tse was a lofty, deep and dignified sage, while Chuang Tse resembled an earthy, irreverent and enlightened hippie. Lao Tse had a very stately demeanor; Chuang Tse was more like a character out of an unconventional hip television comedy with his wild and sharp theater-of-the-absurd perspective.

Lao Tse

Lao Tse (Laozi) wrote the *Tao Te Ching*, translated in English as "The Way and Its Power." After the bible, it is the second most translated book in the world. It was written 2,500 years ago during China's Warring States period. Like the world today, China was in a very confusing stage, which is summed up by the famous Chinese curse, "May you live in interesting times."

Lao Tse passed down the broad tenets of the Water tradition of Taoism, whose principles derived and existed for millennia before his birth. Before the *Tao Te Ching*, they had been passed down through oral traditions. Lao Tse's ideas emphasize the power of yin or softness. He likened the Tao to the empty nature of water that can be everywhere and yet assume virtually any shape or quality while maintaining its essential nature.

His timeless words offer a profound vision of life. He advocated returning to a natural way of living and the spontaneous, easy power of a child. He saw incessant excessive competition as damaging to society, the environment, harmonious human relations and spirituality. He looked at human conflict and war from the perspective of how leaders could smooth, mitigate and circumvent potential damage.

He offered gentle antidotes to pervasive anxiety and the effects of stress on every level. He investigated the roots of and proposed solutions to the lack of personal morality. He has insights into the loss of faith in political, religious and economic institutions that had become corrupt and ineffective. He expounded on the qualities of a teacher or leader and the path of patience and integrity. He felt that the more human beings wanted, the less they could spiritually obtain.

Lao Tse's philosophy had a strong emphasis on personal health, longevity and spirituality. He saw never-ending striving and not following the natural ebbs and flows of life as corrosive to health and peace of mind—especially as we age.

He saw tranquility, naturalness, moderation and keeping the innate soft quality of an infant as the foundations of health and healing. Lao Tse advocated allowing things to happen, rather than making or forcing them to occur.

Chuang Tse

Chuang Tse (Zhuangzi) wrote *The Book of Chuang Tse*, the third seminal work on Taoism. Chuang Tse also emphasized the power of yin, softness and returning to the natural state of a child, but is more well-known for his teachings on spontaneity. He advocated developing the quality of spontaneity until it infuses all actions and becomes natural, even under the most challenging conditions.

Chuang Tse's writing encompasses the most sublime mystical viewpoints, contained within down-to-earth anecdotes and tales. He took the process of spirituality and the Tao very seriously without taking the spiritual process, its followers or himself seriously at all. He irreverently poked fun at everyone's beliefs and judgments—

spoken and unsaid, spiritual and secular. Chuang Tse's wicked sense of humor strongly influenced such seemingly opposite personalities as medieval Zen Buddhists in Japan and twentieth-century Western hippies.

Chuang Tse's aim was to help people avoid the consequences of becoming self-absorbed and rigid. He saw the overly serious or inflexible approach of his Confucian contemporaries as creating all-pervasive judgments that could suffocate the human spirit. He felt this was at the heart of what sidetracked deeper spiritual possibilities. He believed that these judgments did not reflect the true needs of life—spiritually or pragmatically.

As an antidote to pompousness, Chuang Tse emphasized the higher calling of spontaneity and pure awareness over rigidity. He saw attendant investment in "political correctness" and a tendency to repress those who disagreed as fundamental causes of human misery. Nevertheless, he did not advocate that spontaneity should be pursued without regard for others. Being deeply rooted in awareness, he believed, would cultivate the honest spontaneity of a child—without childishness.

Spontaneity and naturalness are the qualities that bagua, tai chi and Taoist meditation practitioners attempt to achieve in their practice forms and daily lives.

A Living Spiritual Tradition

Even though such books as the *I Ching* and the *Tao Te Ching* are well-known, most readers have very little idea about what they mean. They may understand and be fascinated by some of the philosophical principles of these ancient texts. Yet the profound and highly developed tenets go much deeper than might appear from a cursory reading, forming the basis of Taoist meditation.

The Taoist spiritual tradition is about how to completely free the soul or "awaken" as Buddhists might say. Unlike many religions, Taoists do not worship any gods, but instead focus purely on the deeper layers of internal spiritual unfolding within the individual.

TAOISM IS NOT ABOUT SECULAR POWER

Taoism is arguably the only major religion of the world whose practitioners have not sought great secular power. When Taoists took on and acquired such power in the past, it was primarily only out of necessity to correct specific abuses of secular power. When these excesses had been corrected, the Taoists were ready to walk away and freely relinquish their power.

Taoist philosophy considers the outer power structure of civilization, including its politics and economics, to be fleeting and of no assistance to people in their search to find genuine spiritual essence. Taoist philosophy believes these structures simply allow people to go about the business of practical day-to-day living with minimal chaos while having adequate food, shelter and clothing, and so that "the trains run on time."

Inner and Outer Aspects of Taoism

Similar to many religions and spiritual traditions, Taoism has two aspects: the exoteric or outer traditions and the esoteric or inner traditions.

The outer, exoteric branch of Taoism is called *Tao Jiao*. This branch has many of the outward aspects that are commonly associated with religion. It has temples in which Taoists go to pray, seek protection and help from the beyond, consult mediums, have their fortunes told and bury their family, as well as various other services normally expected from a religion.

The esoteric side of Taoism, called *Tao Jia*, has a number of different branches. One of these sects focuses on meditation. In this branch, Taoists seek to find the totality of human experience and the spiritually divine within themselves.

Tao Jia puts the emphasis on each individual personally finding the essence within them. It starts with the essence of themselves and then of the Tao, god-spirit or universal consciousness within. Christians similarly believe that "man was created in God's image," and that God is therefore within man.

This does not imply that humans are gods in the sense that they can physically create universes. Instead, it implies that the source of creation and all the ways in which its energies manifest are potentially contained within the invisible core of each individual. Taoists believe this to be so regardless of whether the individual recognizes it. Through meditation and other practices, we can seek to understand the ways in which the energies that compose the universe exist inside ourselves, as well as discover the nature of existence and humbly manifest it all the days of our lives.

Taoist meditation has various energetic practices that include the transformational practices discussed in Chapter 1 known as *internal alchemy*.[3] These energetic practices lead you to fully understand how you contain within yourself a tiny seed that is identical to the underlying essence of the whole universe. That is, they allow you to realize and embody—in ways beyond intellectual knowledge—the universe that exists inside you. It is only a matter of finding it.

Some say that we can achieve physical immortality through meditation, which is also a goal of Western alchemical traditions. Whether physical immortality is actually possible is unknown, but spiritual immortality is possible. You can awaken and become fully conscious of the potential of your being and thereby free your spirit from the limitations of a human body.

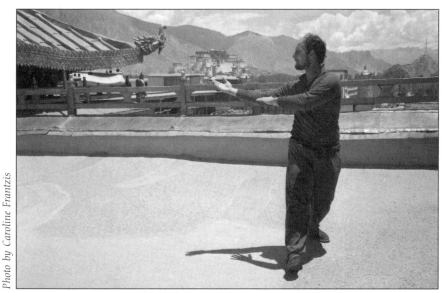

Photo by Caroline Frantzis

The author demonstrates bagua heel-to-toe stepping. This photograph was taken in Lhasa, Tibet, in 1986. The Potala, former palace of the Dalai Lama, can be seen in the background.

---

3 The techniques of inner alchemy, as applied to bagua and tai chi, are discussed in the author's book *The Great Stillness*.

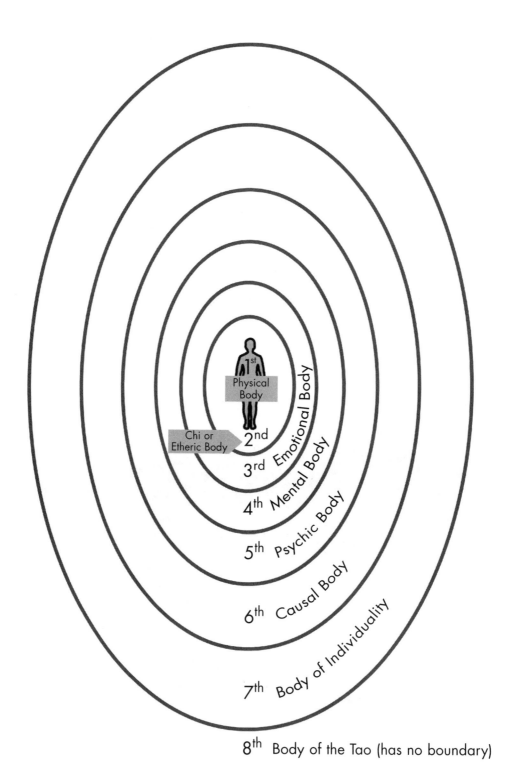

1st Physical Body

Chi or Etheric Body 2nd

3rd Emotional Body

4th Mental Body

5th Psychic Body

6th Causal Body

7th Body of Individuality

8th Body of the Tao (has no boundary)

The Eight Energy Bodies

Eight Energy Bodies

Connected to each of us are eight different energy bodies that spiral into and connect with corresponding energies of the universe.

The eight energy bodies begin with your physical body, which is the densest and vibrates at the lowest frequency of energy. The succeeding bodies consist of progressively more subtle energies that vibrate at higher and higher frequencies. The eight energy bodies are:

1. Flesh of the physical body.
2. Chi body, also known as the etheric body or aura in many Western traditions The etheric body both fuels the physical body and is created by it.
3. Emotional body, which gives rise to positive, negative and neutral emotions.
4. Mental body, which causes thoughts to function with either clarity or confusion.
5. Psychic body, which bridges the seen and unseen worlds. It allows us to find our hidden internal capacities and helps our intuition or psychic perceptions become concrete.
6. Causal or karmic body, which causes karma to flow and manifest.
7. Body of individuality, which enables the actual birth of the full spiritual being commonly referred to as essence.
8. The joining of human consciousness to the whole of the universe or Tao. Few people ever actualize the realization of becoming one with the Tao in any single generation.

Beginning with the physical body, each successive body not only occupies the same space as the previous one, but also extends farther outward toward the stars. Each one is progressively larger than the one before. Your physical body begins inside your bone marrow and extends outward to your skin. Your chi body extends outward past your skin, typically to a distance between two and ten feet, depending on its strength. In turn, your emotional body extends far outside your body deep into space—past our solar system. Each successive body reaches even farther into outer space.

Similarly, each successive body penetrates deeper inside you into what Taoists call *inner space*. In turn, as these depths plunge inside the quantum level within you, they are also simultaneously directly connected to the farthest reaches outside you.

Externally, the eight bodies can be likened to the rings of water that disperse outward when you throw a stone into a pond. Energies flow between and through each of the eight energy bodies. The energy bodies inside connect you to the same energy bodies that pervade all organisms throughout the farthest reaches of the universe.

These energy fields comprise all the aspects that humans can potentially experience regardless of time, place or circumstances. They are in effect maps that enable you to experientially and systematically become aware of the living layers of your consciousness and the chi blockages they each may hold. Eventually, the way your energetic field links you to the energies of other human beings and the universe becomes deeply relevant to daily living.

Resolving Energetic Blockages

Chi flows like a river through you. When free, open and unbound, it arouses positive, life-nurturing forces. However, chi can become blocked or trapped in any of the eight energy bodies. Metaphorically, the river inside you backs up and accumulates sludge and gunk, arousing more negative and destructive forces.

How to become aware of and resolve energetic blockages is the essential practice of Taoist energetic arts, including qigong, bagua, tai chi and Taoist meditation. Commonly, the preparatory meditation practices of qigong, bagua and tai chi, help you become aware of and resolve blockages in the first four energy bodies. They prepare you for the more challenging work of freeing blockages in the higher ones.

Fire and Water Approaches of Resolving Energetic Blockages

The Fire and Water branches of Taoism differ in how they approach energetic blockages. The terms "Fire" and "Water" are metaphors regarding the essential nature of how you engage with specific techniques within the entire range of Taoist practices. This includes all styles and techniques of practice whether or not they have a meditation tradition.

Both Fire and Water branches use some or all of the energetic techniques from the sixteen-part neigong system to resolve energetic blockages in the eight energy bodies. The Water traditions follow more of a yin path while the Fire traditions are more yang.

Water methods emphasize the natural yin process of allowing and encouraging, but not demanding, change. They follow the path of least resistance. Water schools emphasize the twin techniques of Inner and Outer Dissolving to release blockages until the energy of any blockage becomes empty and neutral of all content.

Fire schools emphasize making things happen or consciously engineering them in your inner world. Applications include transforming and controlling energies through conscious focus and will.

In Fire methods, resolving blockages is accomplished by deliberately energetically transforming one quality or attitude into another. An example might be transforming hatred into love, or malaise and paralysis into the capacity for active engagement. Initially, the central focus within the Fire schools is on the microcosmic and macrocosmic (or small and large) heavenly orbits of energy.

Fire and Water methods help you clear energetic blockages. This process eventually leads to becoming conscious of all the physical bodily tissues, and chi and spirit energies that underlie what Taoists call *making the body conscious.*

The Three Treasures: Body, Energy and Spirit

Taoists believe that each of us has three spiritual treasures: our body, the energy that runs through it and our spirit. In Chinese, these are respectively called *jing, chi* and *shen*. The word *jing* literally translates as "sperm," but the concept is that the sperm (or egg) creates a physical body. So jing is the energy of the physical body. Each of these is composed of energy where body-energy is the least refined and vibrates at the lowest frequency and spirit-energy is the most refined and vibrates at a much higher frequency. Chi is in the middle and governs our emotions, thoughts and psychic sensitivities and potentials.

The overarching, initial goal of practicing Taoist meditation is seeking, finding and functioning from the spirit, which is permanent and unchanging. You must guide your spirit to become fully open and clear in order to reach a state of stillness.

For most people, this is not initially possible because the energies at all levels of body, energy and spirit are blocked from flowing freely and openly. For example, poor physical alignments, blood circulation or nerve flow can block the optimum functions of your physical body. Closed down acupuncture points or the inability to store energy in the lower tantien, heart or brain centers (middle or upper tantiens) can block optimum chi flow.[4] Spiritual obstacles might include being excessively self-absorbed, incapable of loving, or fearfully consumed by feelings of alienation, or resentment because of events beyond your control. Any kind of imbalance can prevent you from seeing into the root of your own life and that of existence itself.

External to Internal:
Progression from Body to Energy and Energy to Spirit

All Taoist meditation methods, whether Fire or Water, are also based on three major interrelated, progressive training procedures:

- Development from the purely external to the more and then most internal practices
- Resolving body, chi and spiritual blockages by transforming or dissolving energy
- While continuing to work with the first two methods, digging deeper into the core of your being by exploring the interrelationships among all three treasures

Having a body that functions well is the most external aspect; working with subtle chi requires you to go internal; and freeing your spirit will require going completely internal to the core of your being. Training starts with an external orientation, such as qigong movements, to set the foundation for the deeper, internal meditation practices. If the foundation of any previous stage is weak, work at the next level will normally be less effective and take longer to accomplish with satisfaction.

Moving from the External: Focus on Your Body

All qigong practices can be done standing, sitting, moving, lying down or as partner exercises. Through qigong training you develop your awareness and ability to focus mostly on techniques related to the physical body. Training normally includes some limited chi and spirit work, which fulfills basic needs of the body.

---

[4] See Appendix C for diagrams showing the location of the tantiens.

For example, if you practice bagua or tai chi, you practice until all your physical movements are so natural that you can do them automatically. You're looking for the place where you are attentive without concentrating on every minute detail to perform the external movements. During this stage you must learn to look straight ahead and extend your awareness. You must simultaneously feel your entire body while seeing and comprehending what is happening outside it. You cannot lapse into distracting internal dialogue or space out.

Going Internal: Focus on Chi

Once you master the body practices, your focus shifts to becoming aware of, opening up and consciously directing all the energies within your physical body and external aura. You observe ever more subtle energetic signals, which leads to recognizing tensions in your third and fourth energy bodies (emotional and mental, respectively). The more strongly your chi flows, the easier it is to recognize the spiritual experiences lying at the root of emotional, mental and psychic blockages.

Going More Internal: Focus on Spirit

Here, you learn to feel the internally, exceptionally refined psychic or karmic energies of spirit and resolve the blockages that bind your soul. The most internal levels relate to emptiness and the Tao to which all practices are ultimately meant to take you—if you choose to embark on a spiritual journey.

The Relationship of the Three Treasures to Emptiness and the Tao

As mentioned earlier, the common usage of the three treasures refers to body-energy-spirit. However, that is only part of the story. *Spirit*, in the complete Taoist tradition also implies another two, unsaid stages of emptiness and Tao. In Chinese, the core progression of classic Taoist meditation practice is expressed as: *jing–chi–shen–wu–Tao*. This is body–energy–spirit–emptiness–universal awareness in English.

Evolution of Taoist practice, as represented by this progression, is:

Jing, or physical body (energy or sperm):
- which begets *chi* or energy,
- which begets *shen* or spirit,
- which begets *wu* or emptiness,
- which begets *Tao*—the essential, unchanging root of the universe.

Body includes everything in us that is corporeal, including:
- Gross anatomy and flesh of the physical body (the first energy body)
- The chi that makes the physical body work and enables the physical body to live (the second energy body)
- The energy expressed by the lower, primal animal emotions, such as anger and fear, which is derived directly from our internal organs and glands

Energy in the Taoist classification system includes the third and fourth energy bodies. In terms of the emotional body, the concept of chi also involves sensitivity to higher emotions or the more abstract ones that include feelings over and above the self, such as kindness or love. The mental body encompasses two sides of the same coin. On one side are the lower mental functions of thinking, such as the energy that permits thought to form on a concrete level, for example, "that is a tree" or "this is an open door." On the other side are the higher mental functions, such as the capacity for abstract and analytical thought. Creativity, imagination and, at the most subtle level, direct perception regarding the nature of everything in existence are examples of higher mental functions.

Spirit (or soul) in the Taoist classification system includes the fifth and sixth energy bodies, as spirit more profoundly forms at the energy levels of the psychic and causal (karmic) bodies. By sufficiently resolving the causal body, the spirit grows within the psychic and causal bodies until it breaches emptiness.

The quality of emptiness undergoes refinement until it stabilizes and releases that which prevents you from recognizing the seventh energetic body—the body of individuality, or your genuine essence. Here who and what you genuinely are extends beyond all of manifestation and every self-concept or possible external or internal identity that you have ever had or could conceive.

The progression continues to release the complete potential of emptiness until the Tao reveals itself. This results in what is known as becoming a Taoist Immortal.

Cyclic Nature of the Three Treasures

Once you have a sense of the continuum between the external and internal, you work simultaneously with all three treasures.

You learn how blockages at one energy level can compromise flows in the other two. For example, blockages in your energy channels can deny you full access to the chi of your emotions that run within the same channels. Blockages in your energy channels make it harder to release and resolve negative emotions, such as anger, hate and paralysis. Releasing these blockages will make it easier to replace them with emotions of patience, compassion and the willingness and ability to engage with life. A blockage at the level of your soul, such as spiritual numbness, may inhibit the flow of chi in your liver. This could potentially lead to weakness in the tendons and ligaments of your knees or back.

Recognizing these interrelationships creates opportunities for spiritual awakening. Once you are able to recognize body or chi blockages, you gain access to them and simultaneously can resolve the spiritual blockages attached to them. At the psychic or karmic level, you can unbind blocked chi in your emotions or acupuncture channels and vice-versa, which gives maximum access to your spirit. In circular fashion, you gain yet more access to your body, ad infinitum.

During different stages of development each primary body, energy or spirit practice either increases or decreases the blocking or enhancing potential of the other two. For example, if the goal of your moving meditation practice (such as bagua or tai chi) is to work primarily on an aspect of spirit as you attempt to resolve a specific spiritual blockage, you might focus on a specific single body mechanism. This might include adding specific breath techniques to particular movements or making micro-movement adjustments within your spine, joints or internal organs.

In this way, the energies within these and other affected body parts become access routes. Each leads to nonphysical chi or spiritual blockages that reside in specific tissues within your physical body. Likewise, activating these physical tissues could rapidly afford you direct access to related chi or spiritual blockages. It is a positive feedback loop, and from which direction you will focus your attention is part of the surprise and wonder of the highly sophisticated Taoist energy arts.

The Sixteen Neigong Components and the Three Treasures

The sixteen neigong components are also applied to awaking the energy within the body. Each can be used to amplify blocked energy signatures, helping you become consciously aware of energetically blocked locations. Using neigong can lead you directly and appropriately to the source of your inner spiritual tensions or blockages. Then, the appropriate Water-dissolving or Fire-transforming techniques can be efficiently applied to resolve the source of the underlying spiritual blockage.

Because the three treasures are cyclical, accessing each in turn gives you progressively more access to the next. With experience, as you clear blockages from each of the three treasures individually, you naturally recognize how to approach and resolve the related blockages in all three simultaneously. This sets off a positive upward spiritual spiral through which you slowly but surely release and open your spirit significantly more. Eventually, you might discover stillness.

Finding Spirit

As you practice Taoist meditation, your awareness gradually opens and stabilizes, so that you become comfortable staying in the resolved open free space inside you where pure spirit resides. External and internal pressures no longer lead you to the same blocked and contracted places inside that trigger repeated destructive patterns of behavior or mental churning. You do not need to obsessively scratch old spiritual itches.

In time, you achieve longer periods of stability and function in the new open spiritual space. In a relaxed way, your spirit feels natural and you no longer get caught up in the drama of being stuck, fixated, dissatisfied or elated. These are common experiences when people begin meditating. Once you get past these weak or powerful experiences, you can then experience spiritual relaxation.

Spiritual Relaxation

Spiritual relaxation (*sung hsin*)—relaxing into your Heart-Mind—describes the state of resting in emptiness, which in Western parlance is where the center of your soul resides. Progressively deeper spiritual relaxation gives you the opportunity to open and engage with profound levels of your being or essence.

All the various methods to open the body, energy and spirit empower every level of spiritual relaxation. Increased spiritual relaxation allows you, in ever greater degrees, to recognize and live from your spiritual essence. Your body, chi and thoughts flow deep within and directly into the source of your spirit to settle there.

Connecting to Your Essence and the Tao

When spiritual tensions release and fully relax, your inner world unites. Your inner sense of being that once seemed composed of multiple, separated parts ceases and a stable, indescribable essence emerges. This essence becomes the cornerstone of spiritual living. As the emptiness within nears fruition, answers spontaneously emerge to fundamental spiritual questions, such as "Who am I?" and "What is my place in the universe?" Your unique individual essence becomes obvious and transcends all qualities of personality, personal history and the various internal identities both can engender.

According to Taoist belief, it is only from this level of awareness that truly understanding and eventually walking the path of the Tao—the road that connects all and everything—is truly possible.

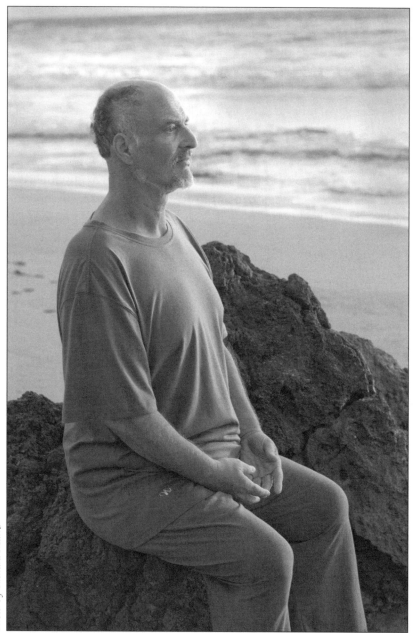

Photo by Richard Marks

The author practices the Inner Dissolving process. All meditation techniques of the Taoist Water method involve dissolving and resolving blockages in the first six energy bodies in order to become internally free.

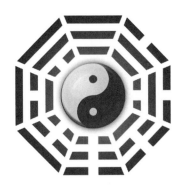

CHAPTER 4
The Relationship of the *I Ching* to Taoist Meditation

Wu Chi, Tai Chi and Yin-Yang

According to Taoist cosmology, before the universe as we know it came into being there existed—and still exists—the undifferentiated void called *wu chi*. Wu chi held within itself all possibilities, but was beyond needing to take form.

However, in order for creation to come into existence, there needed to be a creative force. This force in Chinese philosophy is called *tai chi,* which is the root of the energy practices of tai chi chuan.

When the creative force of tai chi flowed out of wu chi it was—and still is—inherently complete within itself. Yet its method of creation was to separate into two seemingly opposite yet complementary forces: the energies of yin and yang. We know yin and yang today through our familiarity with naturally matched complements/opposites, such as night and day, female and male, dark and light, inside and outside, passive and active.

Yin and yang in turn combined and separated from each other, and transformed back and forth between each other again and again. They formed ever more complex ways of creating and manifesting—the 10,000 possibilities. The interplay between yin and yang continues today, thereby keeping the universe ever-changing and evolving. Within the changing universe, yin and yang continuously partner with each other, within an interconnected continuum, with endless gross and subtle relationships between them.

The Interplay of Yin and Yang

Taoist adepts who developed the essential sections of the *I Ching* used techniques of observation and meditation to explore and experience the entire range of yin and yang relationships. These include the prime energies of pure yin and yang emanating from the void of wu chi. Taoists investigated the highly complex mixtures of yin and yang, which make up the ever-changing infinite phenomena of our visible universe (tai chi).

These adepts deduced that the primal energies of the manifested universe are pure yin and pure yang. To represent these energies, they developed the convention of representing pure yang in writing with an unbroken line (▬) and pure yin with a broken line (▬ ▬).

Most primary energies are pairs of these pure energies of which there are four:
- Yang combined with yang
- Yin combined with yin
- Yin combined with yang
- Yang combined with yin

These can be represented by:

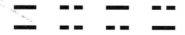

In Taoist philosophy, these four possibilities are called the "four corners" or the "four directions." These principles are also central to the Madhyamika or "middle way," a central philosophy of Tibetan Buddhism to which the Dalai Lama strongly subscribes.

The next level of complexity, which is the basis of the trigrams of the *I Ching* involves energies represented by combinations of yin and yang in threes, which can be represented as:

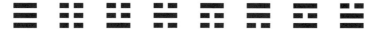

These lines symbolically describe how the upward and downward movement of yin-yang relationships influence, mitigate, enhance and change each other. Yang changes the essential nature of yin and vice-versa.

These combinations are known in Chinese as the *bagua* or "eight trigrams." Taoists identified these energies as the eight primal energies that underlie all possibilities of change. They found that the interactions of these eight energies drive manifestation and change in all other parts of the universe.

Further combinations of yin and yang yield ever greater complexity when applied to the eight trigrams of the *I Ching*. There are combinations of yin and yang in threes, fours, fives, sixes, sevens, eights and to infinitely complex combinations in the sixty-four hexagrams and their connected expansions. Similarly, long chains of zeros and ones in computer code (yin and yang) can be used to create recognizable meanings.

Computer programmers have commented that the complex variables of the *I Ching* presaged modern computer code by millennia. This is because the combinations of the energies of the eight trigrams can be represented as binary code, which involves the use of zeros and ones to represent phenomena. To do so, let yin be represented by zero and yang by one.

The four corners can be represented by:

11   00   10   01

Bagua can be represented by:

111   000   100   010   001   011   101   110

Highly complex combinations would then be a long string of zeros and ones, such as: 111000101000011100001010001101010000101001001110011110101011.

Because the number of combinations is infinite, a universe built from the eight primal energies can also be potentially infinite.

Another key observation that the early Taoists made is that the energies of the universe are dynamic, not static. The energies of yin and yang easily can and do transform into one another. This also includes the fact that they can transform into a state of neither yin nor yang, or both yin and yang. The result is that all the energies that make up the universe—and therefore all of the phenomena that we observe in our world—are also in constant flux. So the world is ever-changing even though phenomena can appear to be constant at a given moment in time. Nothing in manifestation is absolute.

A final key observation made by Taoists is that the interplay and flux of yin and yang at the various levels of complexity is not random. They observed that as the less complex and more primary energies shifted and transformed, all the more complex and less primary energies were affected in predictable ways as well.

Taoists organized their observations into constructs—ways of perceiving patterns or classifications. These served as frameworks, allowing adepts to track how phenomena at all levels of complexity in the universe followed the shifts of the more primary energies. Eventually, these constructs were written down as the essential sections that comprise the *I Ching,* cloaked in symbolic language.

The Sixty-four Hexagrams and the Changing Lines

The *I Ching* is based on all of the ways that the eight trigrams (bagua) or energies of change can combine with each other. These possible combinations are represented by sixty-four hexagrams that contain combinations of yin and yang in six-line combinations. Hence, for Taoists, the *I Ching* is a map that represents how the energy of the universe works. It is a guide to how opposites in the universe—yin and yang—combine, interact and differentiate to represent energy in worlds both seen and unseen by human beings.

Each hexagram can be considered to be a combining of two trigrams with one placed above or below the other.

The Sixty-four Hexagrams of the *I Ching*

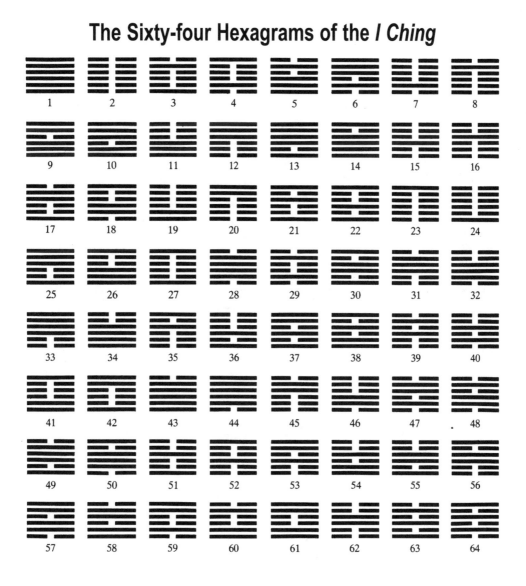

The eight basic energies of change in the universe interact in very subtle ways. Within a hexagram, which combines two of the trigram energies, one of the two trigram energies dominates or is situated over the other. When you mix red paint with blue paint, you do not necessarily get the same purple color every time. A little blue added to a lot of red will look different from a little red added to a lot of blue. The end—manifestation—depends on which energy is dominant and which energy has a mitigating or influencing effect.

When the *I Ching* describes a hexagram as a combination of two energies, it does not necessarily follow that the ratios of the two components are equal. A manifestation described by a particular hexagram may actually embody two thirds of one energy and only one third of the other. Similarly, the combination of the two trigram energies in a hexagram may well be affected by the combinations of the energies of any of the other seven trigrams.

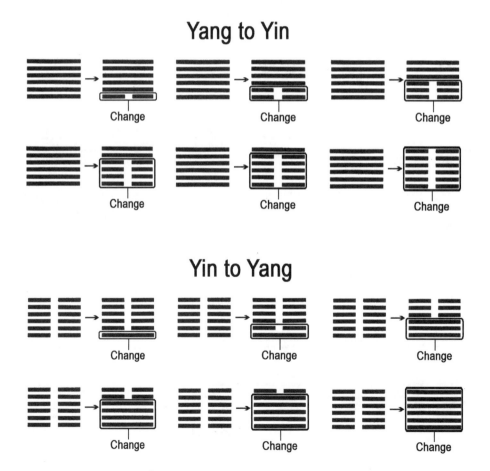

The complex interactions of these energies are in constant flux; nothing ever stops changing. This is illustrated in the *I Ching* by the ability of any of the six lines of a hexagram to change from yin to yang (broken to solid) or yang to yin (solid to broken).

The change of one part will result in changing the entire hexagram. Combinations of trigram energies can also change with similar ease. The effects of such a change can be subtle or dramatic. No matter how the energies interact, change never stops.

Whenever two energies come together or separate, the change itself creates a tremendous amount of energy. The hinge point where energies are either coming together (fusion) or moving apart (fission) is a major focus of the *I Ching* and Taoism. At the exact moment of the separation or combination, the tremendous energy that is released in distinct ways creates very strong possibilities for further change. However, just as this energetic release can be noticed and comprehended it can also go unnoticed or create bewilderment.

According to *I Ching* theory, the morphing of the trigram and hexagram energies, one into the other, leads to change in all aspects of the universe. In fact, the trigrams and hexagrams are not static combinations of the energies, but rather their dynamic qualities and tendencies at a specific point in time. These tendencies are always in transition as they interact and change, divide and subdivide, combine and recombine, and attract and repel other energies and matter. In Taoism, the eight energies (trigrams) interacting in sixty-four possible ways (hexagrams) can be used to interpret all manifestations in the universe, from its vast structures, such as galaxies, star clusters and nebulae; down to their contents, such as the earth and all that it contains—including the smallest forms of life and subatomic particles.

The core sections of the *I Ching* consist of descriptions of each of these hexagrams and their qualities while providing assessments of how the presence of each hexagram's energy is likely to affect and change other parts of the universe. The core sections also elucidate the importance of the different lines within each hexagram. They give insights into the effects that a change in any line—from yin to yang or yang to yin—can have in transforming any one hexagram into another.

By extension, if you understand the map of the *I Ching*, you can learn how the trigram and hexagram energies power changes in all aspects of the universe and your life. A core aspect of all Taoist practices related to the *I Ching* is becoming consciously aware of what these energetic releases—oscillations between yin and yang—might mean and how they can be practically applied. Without such awareness you remain unconsciously affected, like a piece of wood being thrown about by the waves of an ever-flowing ocean of chi.

Intellectual Exploration

Historically, people in China and the West have used the *I Ching* as a philosophical and intellectual tool to explore the nature of the universe and the events of their own personal lives. There are three most common uses of the *I Ching*:

- An oracle for foretelling the future
- A book of wisdom
- A mathematical tool

An Oracle to Foretell the Future

Protocols such as throwing coins or sticks serve as methods to divine the configuration of the hexagram energies dominant in the universe at a particular moment in time. They also foreshadow how and toward what next configuration those energies are changing. The reader then tries to interpret and follow guidance provided in the *I Ching* for how to act in accord with those energies. The purpose is catching larger, universal flows, usually for some personal benefit.

A Book of Wisdom

The *I Ching* passages that describe the qualities of the hexagrams and provide guidance as to how to act in accordance with them offer great wisdom about how events are likely to proceed in the universe. This is true whether in the lives of human beings or the workings of solar systems. For centuries people have used the *I Ching* as an introspective mirror of the events and conditions of their lives. They have used its profound philosophy to delve into, interpret and guide their deeper needs, motivations and actions.

A Mathematical Tool

Another primary use of the *I Ching* is as a mathematical, numerological and diagnostic tool for certain Chinese arts, which focus on flows of invisible energy. These arts include some forms of Chinese astrology and feng shui (geomancy).

The *I Ching* and Taoist Energy Arts

The practice of such energy arts as qigong, bagua, tai chi, Taoist yoga[1] and Taoist meditation, provides you with the capability and sensitivity to both directly perceive and engage with the energies of the *I Ching*. This is not done purely mentally or symbolically, but as living, tangibly felt energetic experiences within your body, mind and spirit. Experiences range from the gross energies of our visible physical world to the most refined spiritual energies of unseen realms that connect to our world.

This kind of engagement with the *I Ching* as a living tradition goes beyond exploring it as an intellectual and philosophical text. Accordingly, it serves as a practical guide to experientially exploring universal energies.

HOW LIU TAUGHT THE *I CHING*

Liu Hung Chieh taught me the *I Ching* in three steps: this is what it says; this is what it means; and this is how to experience it within your own body, energy and spirit. I first studied through chi practices and later through integrating the principles learned into all aspects of my daily activities. Liu felt this was the only way for anyone to fully apply the teachings of the *I Ching* for a very deep understanding of the nature of the universe. He felt this was the necessary process of becoming comfortable with change.

As you Walk the Circle, practice a tai chi form or assume various yoga poses, you progressively understand the interplay of change between yin and yang, or what the ancient Chinese called *liang yi* (also transliterated as *liang-i*). You learn how to flow with rather than fight or resist the energies of change.

Yet, on another level, if there is change, there is also that which is permanent and unchanging. Both concurrently pervade all the possible yin-yang changes included within the universal essence of emptiness that can eventually morph and lead you closer to the Tao. This deeper core of the *I Ching* can be explored through your bagua or tai chi practice.

---

[1] Taoist Longevity Yoga™ is the system that the author has developed to teach Taoist yoga, ancient China's soft yet powerful alternative to what is popularly known today as Hatha yoga.

These pragmatic, spiritual perspectives of how Taoist energy arts are related to *I Ching* are not commonly familiar to those outside the inner gate of the living Taoist tradition.

How the Interplay of Yin and Yang Manifests

You engage with the interplay of yin and yang as you Walk the Circle in bagua and continuously change and reverse direction, or continuously move, shift and turn in your tai chi form. The range of yin-yang energy combinations that you will explore is endless. Here are some common examples:

- The way one part of your body (hand, arm, leg, torso and head) moves forward, upward or right, or how the outside, upward force (yang) is balanced by a equal force going backward, downward, left or inside you (yin).
- Either sequentially or simultaneously—from either the same or different body parts—how your chi projects (yang) or absorbs (yin) chi, including sequentially absorbing energy into one, multiple or all parts of your body (yin) in the first phase of a movement. Then in the second phase of a physical movement, how you project chi (yang) out of a single, multiple or all parts of your entire body at once.
- Simultaneously absorbing chi into your spine (yin) and projecting (emitting) it out of your hand (yang). Or again simultaneously either absorbing or projecting chi out of both your hand and spine.
- Sequentially or simultaneously activating your emotional chi within given movements including constituent mini-parts. Matched pairs of yang and yin in the emotional frequencies of energy, such as anger–fear, enthusiasm–depression, joy–grief and hope–dejection, are all examples. Yin-yang frequencies in the mental, psychic and karmic energy bodies and body of individuality (or essence) are also examples.

Learning to Flow with Change

Bagua and tai chi break down internal resistance to change and teach you how to avoid polarization or fixation on any specific yin or yang quality. At the level of perceptions, representative examples of polarization include:

- I do or don't like it or love/hate it.
- The tree is tall/short, wide/narrow or ordinary/special.

- The universe is big, but I am small.
- I can/can't understand.

Inner tensions are inherently created when the mind focuses exclusively on a single polarity, cutting off or excluding others. This in turn distracts your awareness from the universal. Yet, conversely—and this is a funny thing—when you recognize the universal in everything, the potential opposite changes you experience can simultaneously be effortlessly present. They can also comfortably coexist to varying degrees of importance within your mind. At some point in your practice, you find it becomes completely natural for opposites to coexist without strain.

Taoism, Buddhism and some aspects of quantum physics present us with an interesting paradox to ordinary thinking: All of manifestation—in its endless yin and yang relationships—simultaneously exists and doesn't exist. Yes, from a pragmatic perspective, yin-yang qualities (anything in manifestation) clearly do exist. Yet, if you can remain present to the changeless, it can also be said that yin and yang do not truly exist at all.

There is an ultimate sense of simultaneously recognizing both the continuity of changelessness and the seemingly very real yin-yang experiences inside you. You can arrive at a place where all perceptions—regarding what is happening to you now—don't add or detract from where you might like your body, mind and spirit to ultimately arrive.

With practice, you unravel more of your personal stuck places. Many come to the realization that everyone can get stuck on virtually anything and thereby lose contact with the flow of existence. These blockages underlie and destroy inner peace. They may include experiences of life–death, body–emotions–thoughts, feeling that you do or don't understand and ordinary or paranormal experiences.

Simply realizing that you get stuck sets the foundation for resolving these points and merging into the emptiness that lives at the center of the *I Ching*. A practical value of such study is that in all aspects of your life you become comfortable with change. Then you can learn to flow with change rather than resist or be torn apart by it.

More profoundly, human beings eventually recognize, through direct experience, that inherent to change is its power to destroy anyone who does not possess balance, compassion and naturalness. All three are paramount themes taught in all aspects of Taoist philosophy and chi practices.

Exploring the Eight Energies

Taoists believe that the whole of the universe is represented and present inside every human being's body. The mind of a human being is therefore capable of manipulating the eight energies since they exist inside the body. With practice you could take this to the point of intimately resonating with the energies of the universe that are outside your body. Toward this end, Taoists developed meditation methods.

Using the *I Ching* as a practical guide, bagua and tai chi are two methods developed by Taoists for exploring and balancing the eight universal energies within and outside of the body. You start physically with chi exercises, such as qigong, bagua or tai chi, to clear blockages and make the body stable in the first four energy bodies. You progress to more sophisticated movements and meditation methods to clear and balance the energies in the remaining four energy bodies.

As you balance the energies within you, compassion and naturalness follow. By developing the experiential ability to simultaneously delve inside your body and yet directly experience that which is outside of your body, you gain an understanding of universal energies and how they work.

One of the core methods that Taoists developed to actualize these practices is the Bagua Single Palm Change.

More importantly, those who penetrate even more deeply into the *I Ching* eventually discover that which does not change and remains constant throughout the universe. While the eight energies endlessly combine and recombine—going through alchemical transformations and transmutations—the Tao never changes.

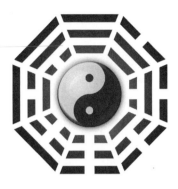

CHAPTER 5
Bagua's Martial and Spiritual Traditions

Bagua has two main traditions. In the West, the better known is its martial art tradition, usually called *bagua zhang.* Less well known is its spiritual or monastic tradition.

Taoist Monastic Tradition

Over time, pieces of the story of the possible origins of bagua as a spiritual tradition have emerged. One of the most intriguing involves a Taoist temple in the south of China: Dragon Gate in Jiangxi Province. Monks there have been practicing the Single Palm Change for 1,500 years. They do this purely as neigong or an internal energy cultivation exercise and spiritual practice rather than as a martial art. This monastery also has records of bagua coming from Shansi Province in Northern China. In Shansi, other records reveal that bagua comes from the Kunlun Mountains, which are north of the Himalayas.

Bai Hua, the disciple of my teacher Liu Hung Chieh in the Taoist Fire tradition, gave me this information. Bai Hua visited Dragon Gate temple to verify these reports. Liu saw records in Shansi Province before the Communist Revolution and said the records were subsequently destroyed during the Cultural Revolution.

The Spiritual Tradition of Bagua and the *I Ching*

According to Liu, the Circle Walking practice of bagua developed by monks some 4,000 years ago had four intertwined purposes:

1. Generate a healthy, disease-free body with relaxed nerves and great stamina, which the monks needed for daily work and prolonged meditation.
2. Achieve stillness of mind.
3. Develop and maintain balance internally while either the monk's inner world or the events of the external world were changing.
4. Realize the Tao.

In the monastic tradition, bagua had one primary technique: the Single Palm Change. It evolved from Circle Walking practice.

Various bagua qigong postures serve as preparation for performing the primary exercise itself. You hold your arms motionless in space whether or not the feet are moving. While maintaining the posture, the initial aim is to bring chi from the belly and spine to the fingertips and stabilize the internal alignments of the upper body.

Once the neigong within specific bagua postures has been integrated, the Single Palm Change proves sufficient to allow practitioners to develop and manipulate the energies inside their body, join them with those outside their body and eventually connect directly to the eight energies of change mapped by the *I Ching*.

Circle Walking and Meditation

When you begin bagua as a meditation practice, your primary focus will be on Circle Walking as a qigong exercise. Practice will encompass all the attendant benefits that it provides for making your body healthy and strong. As this occurs, and as a natural development or continuum, the same Circle Walking methods set the foundation that you need for a deep meditation practice.

Ideally, the first stage is to Walk the Circle without ever putting your hands up in the air. This trains your physical body to become stable and balanced. If you add the arm movements from the get-go, you can easily become hyper-focused on external movement. When you only Walk the Circle with your hands down, it is easier to focus on the physical progress of your lower body.

Are you wobbling or stable each time your foot is in the air, when you plant the foot on the ground or shift your weight from your rear to your front foot? How about when you reverse the circle and change direction?

As your balance and stability grow, you vary the speed of your walking. Your goal is to smoothly change direction and speed, or go from movement to stillness and back again—all without losing awareness. The Taoists say that if you can maintain uninterrupted and complete awareness from the time it takes a leaf to fall from a tree and flutter down to the ground, you will be enlightened.

When Circle Walking alone is learned for spiritual purposes, it is commonly practiced for a few months to a year before arm movements are added.

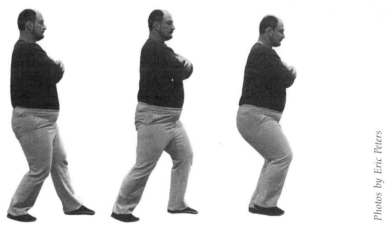

Photos by Eric Peters

The author demonstrates the basic footwork used in Bagua Circle Walking.

Over time, you gradually learn to work with the energies of your physical and etheric bodies. This is done by incorporating some of the basic neigong components, such as body alignments and breathing methods.

As your Circle Walking improves, its value as physical exercise progressively increases. Simultaneously, you develop capacities that are associated with meditation. Through constant repetition, you learn to move the center of your awareness from your head and between your ears into your body, including your feet. You increase your ability to accurately feel all parts of your body simultaneously.

When you Walk the Circle the constant, alternating changes of direction increasingly accustoms the mind to change. For example, if what you visually see outside you constantly changes, your mind gradually and naturally becomes freer and more flexible. It also accepts change instead of becoming fixated and resisting it.

Circle Walking helps you develop a stable center both physically and mentally. When going around in a circle the mind and energy inside you has to become stable, so you don't get dizzy or become otherwise imbalanced. You must progressively let your mind become centered. The goal is to stay with your circling movements and changes of direction without getting distracted by internal chatter or what is happening around you.

Going round and round the circle will also activate the essential vortex energy that lies between the earth and sky. If consciously engaged, this spiraling energy begins to activate, which allows the inner blockages inside you to release. It takes everything that is essentially blocked—physically, energetically, emotionally, mentally and spiritually—and puts it inside a tumbler. Everything shakes up until it shakes loose.

Circle Walking helps you initially explore many key concepts contained within the *I Ching,* including
  • The presence of constant change in the universe
  • The need to retain your balance when presented with change
  • The ability to flow with change and find a place of stillness and balance
    as change occurs.

The Single Palm Change

When you achieve proficiency in Circle Walking, you next learn the Single Palm Change.

As you Walk the Circle, constantly changing and reversing directions, you move your arms and legs in various and unusual ways. These movements and your mind enable you to deliberately align and manipulate the tissues and substructures below your skin. This is practiced in specific ways and is not meant to only imply abstract concepts. You will consciously and specifically direct chi with your mind.

When you direct chi at will, you incorporate into your practice ever more sophisticated aspects of Taoist qigong. You progressively layer into your physical movements more neigong components. Each gradually opens up the body's physical tissues and key energy channels within your body and external aura. As you apply neigong techniques you can activate, clear and free your emotional, mental, psychic and karmic bodies, and beyond.

Practicing bagua as a qigong exercise will improve your health and enable your capacities for meditation to further expand and deepen. Gradually, you will shift from practicing bagua mostly as qigong to meditation. Even so bagua's exercise aspects will continue to support your health.

At this stage, you go beyond exploring the physical and etheric levels of chi and use the Single Palm Change as your vehicle for exploring more refined levels of the eight energy bodies as mapped by the *I Ching*.

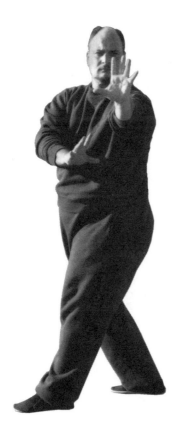 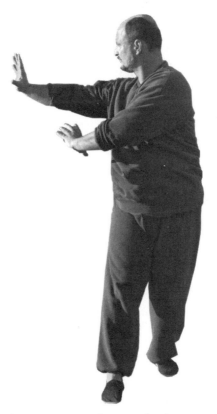

Photos by Eric Peters

The author demonstrates the Single Palm Change posture (front and side views).

The Single Palm Change helps you systematically translate the ideals of the *I Ching* into your daily life. In the early stages you embody some of the *I Ching's* concepts at the physical level. This will in turn motivate you to extend your capacities to other levels of your being.

With the guidance of a genuine master you can physically, energetically and spiritually access, realize and comprehend the nature of the eight energies of change. The Single Palm Change is done in sixty-four different ways to help connect you to the sixty-four hexagram energies of the *I Ching*. Each brings about change from the smallest to the most expansive. If you also learn the experiential methods of using the six changing lines associated with the trigrams, you will find that the Single Palm Change can be done in 312 ways.

The Single Palm Change can be a tremendous personal development tool for discovering previously hidden levels of spontaneity within you. It can also help you smoothly and appropriately respond to life's ever-changing situations. There is an entire art in practicing the Bagua Single Palm Change for relaxation, acceptance that change exists and going with the flow. You cannot fully flow with the universe while you internally fixate or disconnect at any level of your being.

Ultimately, the spiritual practice of the Single Palm Change leads to the place where you have the possibility to recognize that everything is changing and is impermanent except one constant: the Tao.

Cloudy Historical Origins as a Martial Art

The history of the martial art of bagua zhang is obscure. My teacher, Liu Hung Chieh (1905–1986), studied with a man named Ma Shr Ching (also known as Ma Gui). Ma lived and studied with Tung Hai Chuan (1798–1879), also known as Dong Haichuan, the man who brought bagua zhang out of obscurity and into the modern era. Tung is widely credited with introducing the martial art of bagua zhang to Beijing in the mid-1800s.

Tung would never say where his bagua came from. He lived in Ma Shr Ching's house and, in all of the many conversations that Ma had with Tung, he could never get him to reveal the origins of his bagua. Neither could any of Tung's other students.

When I was in Mainland China, I, along with the people I knew, heard and read many popular historical accounts that made all sorts of claims. Each had theories about the origins of bagua, but none of them had sufficient substantiation to be considered fact. According to Ma Shr Ching, Tung Hai Chuan was adamant about not saying where or from whom he learned the art.

In the mid-1980s, I talked to a number of bagua practitioners in Beijing in their eighties and nineties who had known original members of the bagua school. They made it clear that Tung was consistent in his refusal to state the origins of his bagua. Given the circular nature of bagua, in some ways it seems fitting that Tung gave circuitous responses to pointed questions about bagua's origins, such as:

Q: Where did you learn bagua?

A: I learned bagua in the mountains.

Q: From whom did you learn bagua?

A: I learned bagua from a Taoist.

Q: What was his name?

A: He was a very old man.

Q: Where did he come from?

A: He lived in the mountains.

Tung's background is almost as cloudy as that of bagua. He had studied many martial arts in his youth; that much is clear.

However, there are many contradictory accounts about his activities and character during the period between his youth and his arrival in Beijing. Some stories have described him as having been a bandit, murderer, thief, eunuch or pimp while others depict him in much more benevolent terms.

Whatever his character, prior to his arrival in Beijing he seems to have been injured very badly. Tung is supposed to have met a Taoist (or possibly two) who helped him recover and subsequently taught him bagua.

However, all that anyone seems to know for certain is that he showed up on the scene in Beijing, became very famous for his fighting ability and passed on his bagua to a relatively small number of students, seventy-two, all of whom are listed officially on his tombstone.

During more than a decade in China, I had many friends and colleagues who had an interest in bagua that bordered on the fanatical. They had practiced and researched bagua for many decades. Between them, they had met many, many people over the years, and all concluded that there is no currently verifiable accurate historical data about where bagua came from before Tung Hai Chuan.

Today, many people in China are researching the origins of bagua, including the Bagua Association of Beijing and the Colleges of Physical Education in Beijing, Shanghai and Nanjing. There are many theories, but from what I learned in China, no one is willing to bet that his pet theory is absolutely accurate.

Much of the uncertainty about the origins of bagua has resulted from the fact that its history has been handed down solely by oral transmission.

Liu's Experience with Bagua Traditions

My teacher Liu was fortunate to study bagua with disciples of both the martial art tradition of Tung Hai Chuan and the Taoist monastic tradition. During his teens and twenties in Beijing, Liu studied with many of Tung's students and grand students. He studied with Taoist bagua spiritual practitioners when he lived in Sichuan Province during his late thirties and forties.

According to Liu, one of Tung's methods was to teach each student different palm changes or specific variations that would build upon their individual backgrounds in martial arts as well as their other skills and capacities. Tung might teach two different people the same palm change, but with different martial art techniques. He would also teach some, but not all students different aspects of Taoist meditation, about the nature of the mind and the chi within it.

As a result, many of Tung's students came away with varying pieces of Tung's martial and meditation systems. Sometimes groups of them would try to piece together the martial and meditation tradition. This was happening in Beijing when Liu first started his study of bagua, so he was fortunate to be exposed to a broad cross-section of what Tung had taught to his students. The person who mentored Liu in Tung's methods of meditation was named Ju Wen Bao.

When Liu spent ten years in the mountains of Sichuan, he studied in places where and with people for whom the monastic tradition of bagua had continued unbroken since it was said to have been brought from the Kunlun Mountains millennia before. Through such study Liu realized that the meditation tradition he learned from Tung's students was substantial, but incomplete. He was able to complete his study of the spiritual tradition there, which he taught me in tandem with Tung's meditation methods.

Other Bagua Palm Changes

As a young man, I was immersed in palm changes that are practiced within different martial bagua styles. Some schools teach what are known as the Eight Mother Palms; others teach sixty-four palms; and still others teach even more palms. Yet all these schools derive from the martial orientation of the students of Tung Hai Chuan.

In bagua's monastic tradition only the Single Palm Change is practiced. It is about chi, exercise and meditation. In this one simple movement, which has many variations, you can do everything you need to explore the eight trigram energies of change within the *I Ching*. Rather than focusing on a lot of different external movements, you zero in on internal changes, physically, energetically and at all other levels of your being.

I've taught bagua to thousands of people from the perspective of exercise and meditation. I observe that many students like to learn an incessant amount of movements, but often the myriad of movements lack real content.

Most people simply don't have the time to learn a multitude of movements and practice them well. So the majority of students gain the most benefit from a practice that has less rather than more movements. My first bagua teacher Wang Shu Jing advised, "It is better to do one thing well than 10,000 things poorly."

Those who are oriented toward the martial arts and learning many palm changes might keep in mind that the essence of the internal power of the entire bagua martial art system is included within the Single Palm Change. This was illustrated by the way Tung Hai Chuan taught Shr Liu, one of his favorite students who lived with him for a while. In the first six years of Shr Liu's training, Tung only taught him the Single Palm Change with a legion of its internal energy changes and the mental intent of how they were applied in combat.

THE AUTHOR'S EARLY EXPERIENCE OF BAGUA

In my early life, I was exceedingly uncoordinated and lacked a natural awareness of movement. Through training I gained a sense of how to move my body, mostly from practicing martial arts, some gymnastics and free-form dancing. In all of these movement arts, there was almost always a feeling of starting and stopping; you started a move and you finished a move. You did something and then you did something else.

However, when I studied aikido in high school and again in college in Japan, there was more of a sense of flow. Yet aikido itself didn't really flow from one thing to another, to another, to another as a smooth continuum for long periods of time.

When I transitioned into practicing bagua, there was something entirely different. While Walking a Circle there was a profound sense of never stopping, of always making circles and spirals. When practicing, the object was to figure out how to join the natural end of the previous movement with the next movement or with the next palm change. At least theoretically, there was no stopping.

The circles and the spirals in bagua felt somewhat unique, as was this walking in a circle and constantly changing direction. I had practiced spinning techniques elsewhere in other martial arts (karate, judo, jujitsu and Japanese live blade sword) or when gyrating on the dance floor. None of these practices gave me the experience that I got in bagua of going from one direction to another to another to another, so that sometimes within fifteen seconds I changed direction thirty to forty times.

There was a sense of continually being able to turn one way and then the other again and again, and yet have a connective thread through the movements. Rather than feeling, "I'm turning this way," then "I'm turning that way," it was all part of a single continuum.

At the beginning of my practice of bagua, this continuum of movement very much felt like it came from outside my body, from the twisting and turning of muscles. Practicing continuous motions where you never stop, constantly twisting and turning both your arms and your legs, is not done in most movement arts.

Over time, I started getting a sense of internal movement. I began to feel that an arm moving or a leg moving wasn't being generated from my arms or legs, but from my liver, spleen or stomach. I not only had the sense that everything inside my abdomen had become completely alive and was moving, but that the movements everywhere in my body were being generated from inside my belly. This was radically different.

Equally surprising was that even though I felt no physical tension, my body was getting as much or more of a workout than it ever got with the tension that had always accompanied previous training. That tension seemed a necessary part of other martial arts, gymnastics and dance, but it wasn't the case with bagua.

Next, I started feeling subtle energies that the Chinese call *chi* moving in and out of my body: up, down and all around. This had never happened to me before—period. Even when I practiced aikido, I might get one big, large flow of energy, but I never felt the eddies moving between my organs, up my spine, going here, there and everywhere that I got from bagua in ways that were very clear and distinct.

Then, every once in a while, my mind and everything inside me would suddenly become still and extremely quiet, almost as though I was in the eye of a hurricane—a suspension zone. It also was quite noticeable that the more my mind became still inside, the more my body externally started moving at an incredibly rapid rate. This was a totally different experience from any other sort of movement arts that I had encountered.

These profound experiences became the beginning of my exploration of bagua as an *I Ching* meditation art, which I still practice with wonder today—more than forty years later.

This worked with Shr Liu because Tung knew that the physical movements are only a container for the chi and the mind that motivates them. After understanding and embodying the internal energy changes of the Single Palm Change, Shr Liu could perform the self-defense methods of bagua relatively spontaneously. He focused his attention on manifesting the movement of chi and his mental intent through his body.

In contrast, Tung taught most of his other students many, many palm changes. They may have arrived at the same place as Shr Liu, but they did so with an emphasis on physical coordination, internal power training and a lesser overlay of chi.

Perspectives of Three Masters

While training in China with three great bagua masters of the late twentieth century, I always asked them: "What do you think the Single Palm Change is really all about?"

Wang Shu Jing

I remember asking Wang Shu Jing this question after training with him intermittently for around ten years. We were sitting in his home in Taichung, Taiwan. I asked, "What is the most important consideration in bagua?"

"First and most important is the footwork," Wang said. "Other than the footwork, a lot of what is extremely important, you could also understand from doing hsing-i chuan (xing yi quan). Of course, the Single Palm Change is the foundation from which everything in bagua comes. Lacking this foundation, nothing else of real value in bagua can emerge."

Then I asked, "What is most important about the Single Palm Change?"

Wang replied, "There are many things. Of course, your posture and the energy of your lower tantien should always be considered. The Single Palm Change's outer movement is by its nature very expansive. It goes out, your arms go out, your body goes out and these movements have to be intimately connected to the way the inside of your body condenses, so that your chi does also."

He continued, "There must be a connection, a link, a flow-through, between how the chi inside your body becomes very condensed and the chi being able to express itself in an expansive way outside your body through your arm movements. This is the one thing that you should always consider and remember because the power in your Single Palm Change, and the ability to truly have your hands change from one position to another, is completely dependent upon maintaining this link."

After that conversation, Wang gave me his practice sword that hung above his bed. Unfortunately, it was taken from me by a custom's official at Tokyo airport on my way home to America. I made the foolish mistake of not packing it inside my bags because it was not a live blade. The official who took it away said it would arrive with my luggage, but of course it did not. This was a sad event as Wang's gift of the sword was a truly symbolic gesture that was quite heartfelt.

Hung I Hsiang

When I trained with Hung in the 1970s, he mostly taught the first few lines of linear bagua, not the Single Palm Change. He knew I practiced the Single Palm Change because he saw me do it. At the odd moment he would show some movements from the Single Palm Change, but he always returned to the linear bagua. Why he did this, I can only speculate.

However, after classes Hung and his students would commonly go outside onto the streets of Taipei, eat watermelon seeds, drink tea or juice, talk about martial arts and socialize.

One night I asked, "I've read that the most important thing is the Single Palm Change. How do you, Master Hung, see it?"

Hung then said, "There are a few things about how I see the Single Palm Change and its main point of Walking the Circle. First, it is an incredible way to open up the chi inside your body, just as people do with hsing-i's techniques of *pi chuan* (chopping or splitting fist) and *san ti* (power development done standing still and holding the pi chuan arm posture), which we practice almost every night."

He continued, "The Single Palm Change is a powerful method to explore and enable your mind, chi and body to strongly link together. You can do the same thing walking in an even progressively stronger way than is possible by standing still with san ti or doing the simpler steps of hsing-i with Pi Chuan. I would say that this is probably a main point."

"Another point, either in terms of linear or circular bagua, is that I can't really teach so much about how to develop chi. It's not my specialty or nature to communicate that. The way I teach you about chi is how to use it in linear bagua's fighting applications," Hung explained.

In this sense, Hung was very much the opposite of Wang Shu Jing, who always came from the perspective that it was the chi that produced the fighting applications and not the other way around, as Hung believed. Hung's position was simply much more about how to use chi within the techniques of martial arts applications.

Hung added, "Just as practicing linear bagua, when you perform the Single Palm Change, a major emphasis should be on maintaining your centerline. You need to be aware of whether your hands are physically on it. You need to appreciate how you work all the angles that are inherent in the sphere of the Single Palm Change. Over time, it is important to eventually recognize how every angle can change and flow one into the other and how, when you walk in a circle, this moves the inside of you to cause your fighting angles to either freeze or usefully open up."

This piece of advice was not contradicted by any of the bagua adepts that I met in China.

Liu Hung Chieh

When I asked Liu about his take on the Single Palm Change, he would preface his statements by saying he agreed with the points made by Wang and Hung.

"As the Single Palm Change is a big subject, to reasonably answer your question requires that it be looked at from several different perspectives," Liu explained.

He went on to say that when first practicing bagua the main purpose of the Single Palm Change is to get the tips of your fingers, the tips of your toes and everything in the middle to become integrated. When everything is completely connected and flowing through each other, the chi that comes out your fingers, palm, toes, soles of your feet and everything else in the middle of your body becomes one totally unified entity.

Next, the focus is on opening up your body's three tantiens, all the body's main energy channels and many of the smaller ones.

A major function of the Single Palm Change is to create a genuinely stable mind, whether you wish to use it to promote your physical, mental or emotional health, or use it for fighting or meditation. A stable mind is required if it is to be free of anxiety and concerns, and avoid becoming frozen. Without stability, the mind cannot be completely open and free, nor have the ability to move and change between anything—regardless of what that "anything" is.

When the mind is not open and free, it easily becomes frozen (stuck) to varying degrees. This then renders the mind, body, emotions and anything else incapable of being able to freely change and reach its natural conclusion. This applies both to a fighting technique and to what is going on in your inner or outer environment.

A major obstacle that keeps people from understanding the *I Ching* and the Single Palm Change is that they become habitually fixated and stuck. So when anything reaches its natural conclusion, they cannot simply flow into what makes the most sense for where the motion of the universe is going next.

If you look at the Single Palm Change from a martial perspective, along with the unified connection between the tips of your finger, toes and everything else—as Hung I Hsiang said—you need to understand and find out how every single inch of your body can continuously rotate like a sphere. This is what enables you to create and use every fighting angle that potentially exists.

Liu said, "This is why is you must continuously learn many techniques, principles and applications. In this regard, I will teach you many new techniques related to various palm changes. The next step, however, is to become able to make all their essential aspects condense into your Single Palm Change until they settle into your body. No matter how many palm changes you know, they become only a Single Palm Change with many faces."

Liu clarified, "You practice until you recognize that there are not a hundred changes or hundreds of appearances of change, but actually only one. Until, through walking and the Single Palm Change, this reality can stabilize inside you so the one and only change can manifest—even as you change the energy of any martial application within the flicker of a thought. By moving your finger a fraction of an inch, a tiny little bit, all of a sudden, from what is inside, you can do any martial art change that exists and it will jump out of you spontaneously as a fighting application."

"From another perspective," he offered, "the Single Palm Change is also about what I've always considered to be most important for you. It is about more than the chi of your body, emotions and thoughts. Your body already has a fair amount of chi and no doubt it will grow over time. A larger subject of the Single Palm Change is learning about the chi of the spirit and emptiness—to understand the chi that enables you to know who you are, so eventually you can understand the nature of the universe and all that moves within it."

Liu explained, "Somehow while looking at your finger, while moving your feet and body during the Single Palm Change, you join not just with every internal mental state you have, but with Taoism's ultimate purpose of Circle Walking to join your movements with those of the universe. These include the chi of the stars, earth and everything else. As practiced in monasteries for thousands of years, it can be done solely through practicing the Single Palm Change or by sitting quietly in meditation."

"This is why both monks and Taoist Immortals didn't think you needed to do much more than this to achieve the spiritual aims of our tradition. If through one movement you can join yourself to everything in the universe and experience how the universe is moving through you, what more is needed?" he asked.

"The basic spiritual Single Palm Change always begins with the *I Ching's* Heaven Palm," he said.

"Why?" he asked rhetorically.

He answered, "What is not under heaven? Is not the earth part of heaven? Is not the earth part of the universe? Is not the water? Is not the wind? Is not the mountain? Is not the lake? What is not a part of heaven?"

He continued, "Yes, we [Taoists of the Water method] have different ways of doing the Single Palm Change. Still, it always begins with the Single Palm's Heaven Palm and it always returns to the Heaven Palm after moving through all the others. But at the end, there is still only one palm just as there is only one universe, just as there is only one Tao" he said.

He ended with, "I hope I have answered your question."

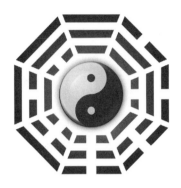

CHAPTER 6
The Art of Tai Chi

Even though tai chi, like yoga, is becoming popular in the West, few know the art's potential. What many see is sequences of movements with one flowing into another. Arms and legs move simultaneously in various directions: up and down, forward and back, right and left, outward and inward. Each movement carries the body into a particular posture from which it then streams into the next.

Observers might think tai chi's silent, fluid and slow motion movements are some sort of sophisticated dance or slow exercise. Indeed a high degree of balance and coordination is developed through practice. It looks so peaceful and relaxed that some might assume it has something to do with meditation. However, if you look more closely you might also notice that its graceful movements resemble kicks, punches and chops.

All these observations are accurate. Tai chi is a martial art, health exercise and a form of meditation.

Like anything that has stood the test of time, there is a lot more to tai chi than what you might gather from first impressions. Tai chi contains important parts of the accumulated wisdom of the ancient world. It can also help you overcome the ever-present difficulties of the human condition and engage with life positively.

Roots in Taoist Philosophy

Tai chi chuan (taijiquan) is the full name of what many people simply refer to as "tai chi." It is composed of two separate ideas. Tai chi encompasses Taoist philosophical and spiritual concepts while *chuan* literally means "fist" or "boxing," encompassing its martial arts or warrior aspects.

Tai (pronounced like the "tie" in bow tie) literally means "large" or "great." The word *chi* (pronounced like the "gee" of gee whiz) is not the same word as chi—internal energy—and instead connotes the superlative of a word, such as biggest, richest or deepest. So tai chi literally means "the maximum biggest," and is often translated by variations on the same theme such as "the supreme ultimate" and "the grand supreme."

Tai chi as a philosophical term is drawn from Taoist's core principles of yin and yang, as well as the balance and integration of the two. From many Western perspectives night–day, up–down, strong–weak, right–wrong, man–woman connote pairs that are in opposition to each other: Something must be either "this" or "that." From an Eastern perspective, opposites naturally complement rather than conflict with each other.

As explained in Chapter 4, yin and yang derive from a common, undifferentiated source that is beyond dualistic opposites called tai chi. Tai chi is the force that brings forth the energies of creation and is the source or cause from which yin and yang separate into the two seemingly opposite yet complementary forces or energies.

At a deep human level, the philosophy of tai chi represents the capacity to balance and integrate any set of opposites within you so that they work with rather than against each other. This includes everything from the mundane to the spiritual. Philosophically and spiritually, tai chi represents the path to personal enlightenment. Wu chi is the path to universal enlightenment.

To implement the philosophical and spiritual possibilities of tai chi you need a method—hence the fluid movements of tai chi forms.

The Martial Art Practice

Tai chi chuan was originally developed in China in the 1600s as a very effective fighting art that drew on Taoist philosophy, Traditional Chinese Medicine and qigong techniques.

Although the *chuan* of *tai chi chuan* literally means "fist" or "boxing," by extension it describes martial arts techniques: anything involving self-defense, warfare or strategic encounters of any kind. Adapted from some of the best techniques of fighting kung fu, the Taoist aspects of tai chi chuan mold and mitigate the aggression inherent in martial arts.

Tai chi is known as an internal martial art because it derives its power primarily through the development of internal energy, as taught through neigong. Tai chi does not develop internal power through increasing external muscular strength and physical tension. These energetic abilities exist independently of self-defense movements.

Like bagua, tai chi's training methods are different from external martial arts, such as karate, tae kwon do or even many types of sports. Tai chi is systematically based on developing the mind, energy and intention. Hallmarks include: sensitivity rather than brute force; muscular relaxation instead of tension; and a calm, still mind rather than a violent, aggressive one. In the martial arts world, these qualities give bagua and tai chi a more spiritual tone than most other martial arts.

History of Tai Chi as a Martial Art

The origins of tai chi are clouded in legend. A popular story is that around the twelfth century, the Taoist sage Chang San Feng (also transliterated as Zhang San Feng) watched a battle between a crane and a snake that inspired him to create some form of tai chi.

More historically verifiable is that a style of tai chi was established in the seventeenth century in central China's Chen Village where its techniques were closely guarded from outsiders. In the nineteenth century, however, an outsider named Yang Lu Chan, posing as a deaf mute, was hired as a servant by the village's most important tai chi master. Working secretly at night, Yang learned and became adept at the form. When he was caught, out of jealousy the other members of the village demanded he be executed. Yang, with the chief tai chi master's consent, challenged his would-be executioners and defeated all of them. After a grueling three days testing his character, Yang was accepted as a student by the master.

Yang then traveled throughout China challenging the country's best martial artists and became known as "Yang the Invincible." He eventually found his way to the imperial capital, Beijing, and taught the imperial guards as well as many aristocrats. He adapted the Chen Village tai chi for his students and created what became known as Yang style tai chi.

From this time onward, distinct styles were developed within specific families and were named after their founders: Chen, Yang, Wu and Hao are the most prominent examples. Each style has a series of distinct choreographed movements called forms, with short ones lasting only for a few minutes and the longest nearly an hour. Each style has many variations and subgroups.

Originally these forms were called solo forms because they were designed for people to practice by themselves. They were developed by the martial art founders of tai chi as a way of training a practitioner's body and mind to acquire certain physical and energetic capacities. Then other training methods such as Push Hands and sparring, where practitioners tested their ability to apply the martial skills developed by the solo forms in interactions with others, were learned.

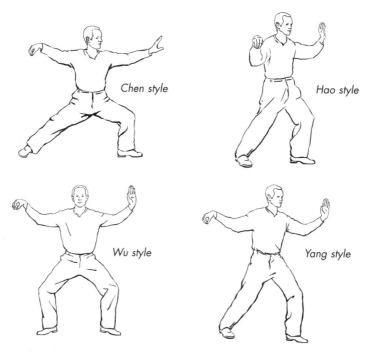

Chen style

Hao style

Wu style

Yang style

Single Whip is a distinctive posture found in most forms of tai chi.
However, this movement is practiced differently in each of the four main styles.

Health Art

Tai chi forms are generally done in slow motion and in very specific ways to relax the body by releasing the nerves and stress in the body. The goal is to be comfortable while getting all the exercise you need to become vibrantly healthy.

Tai chi is the national health exercise in China. More than 200 million people there practice tai chi daily without engaging in any of its martial aspects. Everyone in China has a relative, friend or coworker who regularly practices tai chi. The Chinese know it is incredibly good for health; no one has to tell them.

While living in Taiwan during my twenties, I often encountered Chinese elders who politely asked why I was in China. When I told them I was practicing tai chi, there was usually a concerned look as they solemnly asked in broken English, "What kind of sick you got?"

In China, tai chi was particularly well known as a longevity exercise for elders wishing to regain the functionality and vitality of their youth. Today in China, half of all participants take up tai chi between the ages of fifty and seventy, when the need to overcome the potential negative effects of aging can no longer be denied.

Millions of people in the Western world also practice tai chi to acquire such practical health benefits as reduced stress, improved circulation and balance, and lower blood pressure. Others practice it to enhance their physical and intellectual capabilities.

Competition athletes use tai chi to improve their reflexes and reduce the time it takes to heal from sports injuries. Tai chi helps middle-aged people cope with the ever-increasing responsibilities of life, reduces anxiety and provides a competitive edge in business. Still others use tai chi to develop inner discipline, open their heart and mind, and unleash their spiritual potential.

You do not have to be a martial arts master to gain tai chi's benefits. Nor do you have to be classically fit, athletic or intelligent. Unlike many exercise systems or sports, one of tai chi's most valuable aspects is that it can be done by anyone who can stand up. It even has specific adaptations for people confined to wheelchairs or who can't stand for more than a few minutes. You can practice tai chi if you are overweight or thin, healthy or just out of bed after major surgery, young, middle-aged or very old.

Taoist Qigong Practice

During the first months of learning tai chi, you focus on learning the physical movements: how to move and coordinate the arms, legs and torso, the directions in which to turn and all the details to do with practicing the external form. Unlike bagua, which only has a few movements, even the shortest of tai chi forms involve some ten to twenty or more movements. In addition, you must learn the transitions from one move to the next.

The ideal scenario is to learn principles of body mechanics common to qigong and other energetic practices alongside tai chi. These include
- Physical alignments
- Turning from the waist without injuring your knees
- Keeping the tops of your shoulders down and moving from the shoulder blades
- Many specific techniques aimed at loosening your body, strengthening the internal organs and helping to relax your nerves.

Qigong practice, of which tai chi is a form, provides a foundation for learning and integrating some or all sixteen neigong components. One of the most important aspects is studying how to recognize and develop chi in the body, which involves releasing energetic blockages.

However, the ultimate goal of tai chi as a qigong practice is to optimize hundreds of important yin-yang relationships within you. You are engaging in a process of making your body conscious. By putting the mind inside the body, you tune the mind so it becomes conscious of all the gross and subtle movements of energy within it. Learning to separate any pair of specific yin-yang relationships into their constituent parts develops the potential of each while coordinating and maximizing the smooth flow between many individual pairs of opposites. The yin-yang functions are then integrated within your entire body and being, which empowers you to grow stronger and healthier as a whole.

THE MIND CONTINUUM OF BAGUA AND TAI CHI

Because they are so closely related, the mental frames of bagua and tai chi are often confused, so some people inappropriately practice bagua like tai chi and vice-versa. Consequently, many fail to get the most out of what their practice could offer them.

Although both arts seek to work within a smooth mental continuum, where the qualities of yin and yang are ever-changing, bagua and tai chi have different methods for actualizing them in your body, energy and spirit.

In most tai chi forms, the emphasis is on having a mental continuum that feels as if it has no beginning or end. (The Chen style and other fast forms are the exceptions.) You work to achieve a gradual and smooth continuum where you go in one direction for a while before shifting to another, as if you were lazily moving on a still lake. The mental frame of tai chi aligns with its original Chinese name *chang chuan* (zhang quan) or "long boxing." It suggests the idea of the continuum of China's Long River, which constantly moves for thousands of miles without breaking its flow.

In bagua, you continuously move in an unpredictable path that winds, twists, spirals and can rapidly change from one direction or one technique to another. You often do this in fast and abrupt ways, which could be likened to going downstream through white water rapids or riding a whirlwind.

Even so, the goal is to have the mind's continuing and unbroken intent remain completely smooth. You are meant to keep this stability amidst the physical and energetic changes the body undergoes. This smooth, even, unable-to-be-ruffled center comes from the open place inside all human beings that is eternally stable and never changes. In the *I Ching* it is metaphorically described as the empty center of the symbols for the eight trigrams.

Bagua trains your mind to be very steady regardless of how external events flip from one thing to the next. During Circle Walking your mind eventually develops absolute stability within its dynamic movement. It changes from one thing to another and moves through them without becoming overly anxious or fearful even when the sky seems to be falling.

Bagua's Circle Walking training is meant to take you beyond the fear-greed, hope-fear, elation-depression, emotional-mental swings to which so many are prone in this age of anxiety.

Some aspects of making the body conscious include comprehending how internal energy and the physical tissues of your body work with or against each other. You will also practice navigating the relationships between intent and manifesting chi or physical movement.

As you develop your capacities in these areas, you develop more chi, which is necessary to improve your overall health, boost vitality and longevity, and provide many more benefits that enhance your overall quality of life. Energetic practices serve as a foundation for proceeding into tai chi's spiritual practices, should you choose to do so.

Taoist Meditation

Tai chi forms can be adapted to become vehicles for profound levels of Taoist meditation. Tai chi forms are similar to long qigong sets that have been used by Taoists for thousands of years for exercise and spiritual development through meditation. Many Taoist qigong forms have as many physical movements as or more than tai chi long forms.

During the twentieth century, some Taoist meditation schools adapted the meditation techniques that were traditionally practiced in long qigong sets to tai chi. Only a few tai chi masters I met in the East knew how to apply tai chi as meditation practice. My teacher Liu was one of them.

Like others who knew the practice of Taoist meditation, the tradition would only be shared with practitioners who demonstrated a sincere desire to embark on a spiritual path. Such students would also have to achieve a high level of proficiency in their bagua or tai chi practice.

Concurrently, with learning bagua's Taoist meditation tradition, my teacher Liu taught me how to apply Taoism's spiritual and meditation principles into Wu style tai chi. In my years methodically researching, seeking out masters and practicing in China, I never personally encountered or heard about the meditation methods of long Taoist qigong forms within any other tai chi style.

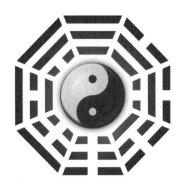

CHAPTER 7
Sophisticated Health Exercises

Throughout history, qigong techniques have been incorporated into bagua and tai chi. They have proven themselves as sophisticated methods that improve and maintain health, reduce stress and increase stamina. Few exercise systems can match their potency and effectiveness. Even as powerful health exercises, each simultaneously trains meditation capacities.

In recent years, tai chi is being increasingly recommended by the medical community as a viable alternative to aerobic exercise for improving and maintaining health. In time, bagua very likely will become part of this mix as the body of practitioners grows and clinical studies can demonstrate its many health benefits.

Western and Taoist Concepts of Exercise

Western paradigms mistakenly lead people to believe that the only way to improve health is through high-intensity, high-impact aerobic exercises. Many doctors and health websites advocate aerobics for strengthening your heart and lungs, using oxygen more efficiently, controlling blood glucose levels and boosting the immune system. Many doctors recommend jogging or bicycle riding for people that have suffered heart attacks.

These ideas persist despite the fact that many clinical studies show that low-impact, low-intensity exercises—such as tai chi—can have the same positive effects on physical health as aerobics or high-intensity sports.[1] Tai chi and other low-impact exercises are as equally effective as aerobics in improving circulation, decreasing blood pressure and increasing oxygen efficiency. Tai chi is extremely effective in improving physical balance in the elderly, a claim virtually no high-intensity aerobic exercise makes.

One of the major values of low-impact exercises is that people of any body type and age can do them without jarring or damaging their joints. Tai chi can be practiced by people who are ill with chronic diseases, including asthma, arthritis or diabetes, which often limits the types of exercise they can do.

Health versus Fitness

Traditional Chinese Medicine has long made a distinction between health and fitness. It defines health as having a state of wellness in which your mind is clear and your emotions are balanced (mental health), your body is free from organic illness or injury, and you experience strong vitality and a sense of well-being.

Fitness is more commonly associated with the superior external performance of high-performance athletics. In the West, a person who is considered to be fit may be able to do one hundred or more pushups, run a marathon, have a beautiful muscular physique and yet not be healthy under their tight abs. He or she may have a bad back, damaged joints, liver problems, unbalanced emotions, an inability to handle stress, lack of libido and other sexual weaknesses. In China, that person would be considered fit, but not healthy.

Conversely, in the West someone would not be considered fit if they looked frail, dumpy or fat, were unable to run a few hundred meters, or did not have physically powerful muscles. Yet that person may be quite healthy. He or she may have a strong back, good joints and blood circulation, be emotionally balanced, have no internal organ or central nervous system problems, engage in all of life's normal activities comfortably and with stamina, have a fulfilling sex life and be able to handle immense stress in a relaxed way.

---

[1] See the website *www.taichiresearch.com* for tai chi case studies.

Thus, you could be considered fit and yet not healthy, or healthy and not fit. In China, the goal is to be healthy and fit: Bagua and tai chi help you achieve both.

WANG SHU JIN: FIT, FAST, FLUID … AND FAT

Wang Shu Jing was my first bagua teacher. I began studying with him in 1968 at the end of my freshman year of college in Japan.

When I first met Wang, he was nearly seventy years old and dramatically overweight. He looked to me in the neighborhood of 300 pounds, a number thrown around very frequently in his later years. Yet he could move fast and fluidly, as if he were in his twenties or thirties. I found this rather exceptional.

After getting to know Wang and seeing and feeling everything Wang could do inside his body, my standard American ideas of what a big fat guy could not do simply went out the window. Here was this seventy-year-old person, huge as a house, who was really strong and who could move like lightning. He seemed almost superhuman.

At the time, I was about 5'10" and a relatively thin 160 pounds. However, in my mid-thirties, I ballooned after a car accident that nearly broke my back. Then in my fifties, I had other car accidents that led to more weight gain. So it was very useful to have trained with Wang to understand that having a big body was not an obstacle to having a good and healthy life.

The Ideal Body

The Western ideal of a healthy person is the Olympian athlete, standing tall and fully muscled. The Taoists' ideal is a baby.

Consider the differences in energy. Who has more life energy? An athlete or a baby? The answer is a baby. Just try to continuously mimic a baby's motions as it randomly moves and plays. It doesn't take long before you become exhausted. The athlete would also soon become exhausted.

Now consider the difference in body types. The Olympian athlete's body is straight, tall and hard. Babies are round, soft and very relaxed. Yet babies are not weak: Pound for pound they have immense yet relaxed strength and stamina. If you're a parent you know how fast babies can wear you out. The more relaxed you are, the more energy you have.

Taoists developed qigong exercises to help people achieve the stamina, relaxation and flexibility of a baby. Qigong shares with Chinese medicine the perspective that health is not determined by the strength of your muscles, but by the strength of your chi. If your chi is abundant, balanced and flowing fully and evenly through-out your body—especially within and between your internal organs—then you will enjoy good health.

Bagua and tai chi make these useful goals accessible to everyone.

Metaphors of Movement

Several analogies are commonly used to describe the types of movement, feeling and sense of the body that are particular to bagua and tai chi. Tai chi is fluid, like water, but rooted like the earth—yin and receptive by nature. In contrast, bagua is like a tornado or whirlwind—yang and male by nature. The bagua body is exceptionally strong and springy, like flexible steel. These are not metaphors rou-tinely used to describe even the fittest of athletes.

A person trained in tai chi is exceptionally relaxed, but completely present and aware. Although bagua practitioners are not as super-relaxed, they are generally considered to be stronger than their counterparts in tai chi.

Training to Optimize and Maintain Health

As exercise systems that provide health and fitness, bagua and tai chi train you in ways that are not common to most other forms of exercise. There are two major reasons.

First, the training methods of bagua and tai chi are designed to optimize all rather than only some of the body's internal systems. In contrast, most forms of exercise focus almost exclusively on developing one's muscles.

Second, a primary goal of both bagua and tai chi is to develop and strengthen energy flow in the body by relaxing the nerves and freeing any blocked or trapped energy within them. These methods are similar to those in qigong exercises.

The Primary Positive Effects of Training

- **Release and relax the nervous system.** Anxiety and stress that leach into most people are due to habits of tension that lie deeply within the nerves of the body. Tension not only defeats relaxation, but also when not released, perpetuates and exacerbates the inability to relax. It's a negative feedback loop.

  Bagua, tai chi and all energy arts train you to stop creating nervous tension in each part of your body and mind. So you can work, play and interact with others from a deep sense of relaxation and awareness.

- **Exercise and tone all your small and large muscles, tendons and ligaments.** The goal is to open up space in your body and exercise everything within those spaces. This makes sure that blood flow can reach all the nooks and crannies, particularly in and around all your internal organs. Blood is the portal that delivers the nutrients your body needs for healing and maintaining wellness. Where there is blood, there is life.

- **Move all your bodily fluids optimally, including blood, lymph, synovial (between your joints), spinal, and the fluids of the brain as well as those within and between your internal organs.** The body works best when it has a constant interchange of fluids in and out of and between all its internal systems.

  Since our bodies primarily consist of fluids, a fundamental principle of bagua and tai chi is getting these fluids to pump throughout the body with a very strong, regular and balanced flow. This allows the body to work optimally and prevents weaknesses, particularly in your internal organs.

  Many exercises that contract your muscles move some fluids well, but not others. They may be great for your cardiovascular system, but may not be as effective for your liver, spleen and kidneys. Bagua and tai chi positively affect the fluid interchanges that occur throughout the body by creating direct internal pressures throughout the body, especially into, out of and around your internal organs.

  Bagua and tai chi train you to move and turn from the *kwa*—also referred to as the bikini fold or inguinal crease—as well as moving your arms and shoulders while keeping the back of your knees and the armpits open.

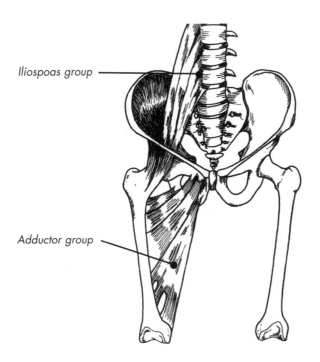

Iliospoas group

Adductor group

**The Deep Muscles
of the Kwa**

These are the areas where you find the majority of the lymph nodes in your body. Bagua and tai chi train you to deliberately increase the flow of lymph, which helps strengthen your immune system.

Bagua and tai chi train you to contract and expand the spaces inside your joints, which strengthens the flow of synovial fluid and helps prevent arthritic conditions.

- **Twist the muscles and other soft tissues as you move.** This facilitates the spiraling of chi and gives you a stronger flow of energy. The twisting of the tissues and muscles in bagua and tai chi simply means that the tissues of the body are constantly turning left and right. Most exercises work on the forward and backward longitudinal movement of bodily muscles and tissues, rather than focusing on the left and right lateral twisting movements as do bagua and tai chi.

Twisting the tissues in the arms and the legs eventually twists and moves the ligaments attached to the spine. Such twisting provides a constant massage of the internal organs and can help to relieve and prevent minor back problems.[2] Back and neck issues are one of the most common reasons for doctor visits.

Twisting facilitates the way that energy naturally spirals through your body. The spiral is the universal movement of all forms of organic life. Natural organisms don't move or grow in straight lines, but rather in spirals. Chi also moves through your body in spirals.

When infants crawl, their arms and legs constantly twist, which is how they get moving. They flip around from their belly or back by twisting the insides of their hips and belly.

However, as children grow older and copy their stiffer, straighter adult role models, they lose this twisting action. This in turn causes them to lose the incredible abundant energy they had as infants. Bagua and tai chi emphasize twisting the tissues and spiraling chi to help you regain such energetic capacities.

- **Increase your body's elasticity.** The human body—contrary to popular opinion—is not held up by bones. It is held upright by a series of ligaments that are actually much stronger than bones. What connects your foot to your belly to your neck is a series of interconnecting ligaments or fasciae that are connected to ligaments.

   Bagua and tai chi train you to release these ligaments and fasciae so that you have as much unrestricted movement as possible. In doing so, they become incredibly elastic, like a rubber band. This quality is found in babies. The next time you encounter a baby, pull their hands, arms and legs (gently now!) and observe this rubber band quality; their limbs are soft and springy. Bagua and tai chi seek to recreate these qualities inside you.

   Elasticity significantly increases the range of motion in your joints, spine and internal organs. It allows optimum movement within the joints and between the vertebrae of the spine. Constant pulling and releasing of ligaments inside your body causes the natural and healthy movement of internal organs. It also massages them and makes them springier. Together these actions enhance blood and fluid flows, which are important factors in determining your health. Most people don't even think about their fluids.

   As elasticity increases, so too does the spiraling of energy. This movement

---

[2] If you have major back, neck or joint problems, bagua is not recommended. However, you can check with your physician to see if qigong or tai chi might be appropriate for you.

causes the joints and spinal vertebrae to constantly pulse so that the spaces within them continually shrink and grow. Pulsing stimulates the flow of fluids inside the joints and between and within your vertebrae. Taoists call this pulsing action *opening and closing*. This rhythmic movement keeps the soft tissues of the joints flexible and elastic.

Arthritis and the loss of mobility and flexibility can make you prone to injury, or harden the ligaments. In contrast, keeping the body elastic and the fluids moving strongly in your joints helps you avoid many of the problems associated with aging.

- **Teach your body to flow.** Bagua and tai chi train the entire body to move in a flowing, coordinated and continuous manner without abrupt starts or stops. These two arts create a smooth continuum of unceasing flow, much like a pendulum. Both promote flow externally in your physical movements and internally within all the parts of your body: organs, ligaments, tendons, tissues, fluids and muscles. Most people start out being very clunky and jerky with their movements: starting, stopping, freezing and beginning again. Bagua and tai chi training helps you to learn how to flow smoothly.

  Ultimately, the ability to find the flow requires that all parts of your body—especially your nerves—be very relaxed. Relaxation is necessary so that the flow of your fluids can be fairly smooth and circulate in an unrestricted way throughout your body. Chi flow in the body must also be reasonably smooth and balanced. This flow rarely comes from pure physical athleticism.

- **Enable whole-body movement.** Almost all athletes want to develop whole-body movement. However, what they're usually after is having the arms, shoulders and torso move together. The whole-body movements of bagua and tai chi are primarily generated from deep inside your body—reaching from the tips of your toes and fingers to the crown of your head.

  Tai chi movements are initiated from deep inside the hips and belly, and move through all the systems from the toes to fingers to head. Bagua movements are initiated from the feet.

- **Make the body simultaneously soft and strong.** Bagua and tai chi train your body to move in any direction completely unimpeded. Your body can become like a piece of silk that moves absolutely smoothly as it flutters in the wind.

Practicing bagua and tai chi can make your arms very heavy, literally with the strength of iron. Yet paradoxically, when they move with almost lightning speed, they look and feel virtually weightless and light.

All these qualities become simultaneously trained inside you as you practice bagua and tai chi. Their positive, regenerating effects are like circles coming in and moving out of circles that increase in size and strength. As your nervous system relaxes, the other body systems connected to your nervous system are continually upgraded, which in turn helps relax the nerves even more.

Aerobic Benefits

Although tai chi can provide you with many of the same benefits as aerobic exercise, it is not normally any more aerobic than ordinary walking. Only when practiced as a martial art, where the training includes Push Hands, fast forms and sparring practices, does it becomes more aerobic.

Bagua, especially where you Walk the Circle at a fast pace, provides all the same aerobic benefits as speed walking or running without the high impact.

For those interested in fitness as well as health, bagua is exceptionally effective. Practicing with fast Circle Walking and frequent Single Palm Changes will strongly work your legs, hips and internal organs. It will also twist, lengthen and strongly exercise the muscles, tendons, ligaments and fasciae of your arms and back. In this way bagua can make you exceptionally fit. You can even put light weights on your arms for resistance training.

However, before you train for fitness in bagua or tai chi, you must first become healthy. If you are exceptionally healthy and fit, then you may use the skills you acquire from fitness-orientated bagua or tai chi to excel in business, athletics, energy arts or anything on which you choose to focus your intent.

Similarities and Differences of Two Arts

When practiced as qigong exercise arts, bagua and tai chi are dramatically more similar than different. They essentially implement the same chi-cultivation techniques, even though they are practiced very differently. Each art involves distinctive body feelings, strategies of thought and philosophical approaches for accomplishing goals. Each has its relative strengths and weaknesses.

The Basic Underlying Principle: 70- and 80-Percent Rule

Common to bagua and tai chi, and all other Taoist Water method energetic practices, is the 70- or 80-percent rule—the rule of moderation. The idea is to neither do too much nor too little. This fundamental principle is also echoed in Confucianism where it is called the "Golden Mean."

In qigong and tai chi, the 70-percent rule is applied as a more yin way of practice, whereas in bagua the 80-percent rule is applied as a more high-performance, yang way of practice. In bagua, 70-percent is applied when you are in average shape and 80 percent after you become very fit and are not suffering from any illness, injury or other physical limitation.

When training in all aspects of bagua and tai chi, this rule asks you to stay within 70 or 80 percent of your capacities. The rule of moderation applies to every aspect of which you could conceive in your practice, such as

- How you practice a certain physical or energetic movement
- How far you stretch or bend your arms, legs and torso
- The length of time you practice
- The attention you place on creating movements or chi flow.

When you stay within 70 percent of your limits, your training will progress at a much faster pace, be more effective and enable your system to more easily integrate what you learn. Only those who are very healthy and fit should practice to 80 percent of their ability.

By applying this rule, the absolute amount (100 percent) of what you were capable of doing when you first began your practice continues to improve and increase upward—smoothly and without strain. As you reach each new pinnacle of health, strength and stamina, your 70- or 80-percent limit continuously trends upward. Most importantly, you avoid the negative effects of overstraining.

This method of practice directly contrasts with many standard Western training methods, which train you to continuously push and go to extremes. Many modern exercise systems ask you to perform pushups, squats or run until you drop. Most professional athletic coaches scream and yell, demanding not 100 percent but 150 percent. This type of training revs the nerves and increases the general levels of tension that lock in your body even after the workout is over.

From the Taoist point of view, the moment you push past 100 percent, you generate resistance inside yourself. When your body and mind severely overstrain or excessively stress, they reach a tipping point. The system rebels and physical or psychological injuries lurk around the corner. The body's defense mechanisms take effect, and you become less willing to physically move.

Keeping a 20- or 30-percent reserve will keep your body and mind from going into stress or overdrive. The rev drains rather than increases your capabilities. Keeping to the 70- or 80-percent rule helps you learn faster while increasing your strength and stamina more quickly than overtraining and overstraining. It ensures that you maintain a margin of safety, preventing injuries and exhaustion.

The excitement in your mind might push you far past your natural physical limitations. In your mind you might move a lot more exceptionally than your body actually permits. So keeping safety first in mind will help you adhere to the 70- or 80-percent rule.

In terms of chi, staying within the rule of moderation helps you continuously increase rather than deplete your chi. Stress and tension diminish chi flow, which is the most important factor in your overall health and wellness.

Moderation helps you become healthy, not only in terms of your body, but also in your psychological disposition. Both attempt to foster good mental health as opposed to obsessive-compulsive disorders to which many athletes are prone.

Injured or Out of Shape?

If you are injured, continuously in pain, severely out of shape or have serious health problems, you should check with your healthcare provider to make sure that tai chi or bagua is appropriate for you, and then drop your training back to 30 or 40 percent or less of your capabilities. If you have constant pain, your goal is to drop back from 70 percent to a point before your pain level escalates to the next higher dramatic level.

A common injury is to the shoulder. If your shoulder or arm is hurt and you feel pain when your hand reaches your nose, your hand should go no higher than your chest. Once your body softens and the pain goes away, you can increase your range of motion a bit more—maybe to your chin. As your hand can go higher without strain, you have a new measure for your 70 percent. You may find that eventually you can even painlessly move your arm vertically over your head or have enough looseness to actually put your hand behind your head.

If you try to push past your pain, as many do, you will not provide your arm with the means to regenerate and completely heal. Instead, you will build tension and resistance, which can result in further injury and more pain. By maintaining a slow, steady progression you actually increase your rate of recovery.

Yin and Yang Manifestations

Bagua and tai chi complement each other as arts within the same family. A powerful synergy is created in the body by combining the strength that bagua's yang energy develops with the extreme softness of tai chi's yin energy.

Bagua starts out with an emphasis on becoming yang—open, full and outwardly directed. In tai chi, the emphasis (at least in the beginning) is to become yin—very soft, round and yielding. At some point, however, both endeavor to manifest and combine each other's yin and yang aspects seamlessly.

Bagua initially seeks to produce a lot of yang energy within you. Yet it is incredibly relaxed yang energy that lacks the aggression and anger commonly associated with yang energy's martial aspects. Likewise, in tai chi, even though you are initially seeking to produce yin energy, this very relaxed yin energy is not collapsed. It is very full, vibrant and eventually creates a core of steel inside it.

My teacher Liu practiced bagua and tai chi until the day he died in his eighties. He said that on those days when his body or mind felt relatively hard and stiff, he practiced tai chi more. On those days when he felt relatively soft or weak, he practiced bagua more.

Differing Speeds of Movement

One of the more important differences between bagua and tai chi is the speed at which you normally move when you practice. Tai chi is commonly done with two kinds of speed. Ninety-nine percent of all tai chi movements are done very slowly, smoothly and evenly. However, even though you move smoothly and evenly, you can move from slow, to very slow, to super-slow almost like molasses dripping from a spoon. Reaching an absolute pinnacle of slowness allows your central nervous system to fully release and become balanced. This allows you, if you so choose, to move with lightning speed at will. It is one basic method of how real speed in tai chi as a martial art is trained. Sufficiently releasing the nervous system makes it possible for your body to move at any speed with virtually no internal resistance.

Only one or two percent of tai chi is done alternating between moving exceedingly slow or fast. For example, this is done in the Chen style and in the fast movement practices of the Yang and Wu styles. The fast parts can be very dramatic, especially when they result in strong, fast and explosive releases of energy.

Bagua moves differently. As a general rule bagua practice is at an easy-going and smooth normal walking pace. Even though you might move with the same sort of fluidity as tai chi, most bagua—at least past the beginning stage—is also practiced between moving fairly quickly to lightning fast.

Once you advance to practicing at fast or super-fast walking speeds, seldom would you practice your movements in super-slow motion. If you do move very slowly, it is only for temporary transition periods. For example, you might need time to assimilate a specific, physical coordination aspect or learn a new movement that you find particularly challenging.

Bagua seeks to release the nervous system, but in a very different manner from tai chi. Most of its movements are deliberately done faster and faster over time and as smoothly as possible. The movement, internal chi and mind internally fuse to release the nerves to the same degree that is done in tai chi by moving in exceedingly slow motion.

Different Sizes of Movement

Generally, in most tai chi styles, the physical size of their movements is determined by whether the specific tai chi style is called a small, medium or large frame style. The sizes mentioned here are metaphors for the relative, but not necessarily the absolute physical size of the movements.

All tai chi movements are supposed to be circular or at least made up of arcing motions, which define the size of their movements. In a small style, a move might be done with circles that are one to three inches in diameter. In a medium style, the same move might be done in a circle five to seven inches in diameter. In a large style, the circle for that move might be ten to twelve inches in diameter. In general, the bigger the typical circles of a specific style's movements, the larger the frame of the style.

In general, the smaller a bagua circle or tai chi style's frame, the more complex are its internal movements. Small frame movements have more extremely subtle and refined turns, circles and spirals hidden within their physical movements. Although the principles of movement are the same, they are condensed into a smaller space. The vast majority—80 percent or more—of all tai chi movements taught throughout the West are composed of medium frame movements. Small frame movements are the least prevalent.

Bagua doesn't distinguish as sharply as tai chi between big and small because virtually every movement in bagua can be done big, medium or small—regardless of the style. However, it is more common for teachers to initially teach bagua movements as large frame movements. Later they typically shrink them to smaller and smaller frames until students can easily flow between each in a seamless manner. Eventually, they can learn to change the size of their motions easily and naturally at will.

Bagua and tai chi strongly emphasize fully articulating the joints in every possible direction. Bagua generally gets the joints to articulate a little more fully than Yang or Wu style tai chi. However, the Chen style of tai chi comes the closest to bagua's degree of working with the movement of the joints.

When to Start Learning

Almost anyone can start and keep practicing tai chi at any age—even the elderly. Tai chi has virtually no limitations on who can begin or continue to practice because it is easy on the joints.

With bagua, seventy years is about as old as you could begin, unless you are very healthy and fit or you have practiced qigong or tai chi for a long time. Your joints (especially in the lower body) and spine must be relatively healthy. If this is not the case, the twisting movements of bagua have the distinct potential to make your joints worse—especially in the knees or spine—when overdone. Nevertheless, if your joints are in good shape to start with, bagua can make them exceedingly strong, much more so than tai chi.

Choosing Your Art by Personality Type

Bagua suits people who like to be challenged. Its vigorous motions tend to attract people who prefer moving fast, have a strong sense of accomplishment, like the internal focus but dislike slow motion. Since bagua places a greater emphasis on faster movement, it appeals to those who are slightly more naturally athletic. As soon as you start bagua, the challenges become very obvious even to the casual observer.

Bagua is particularly useful for people who have a very passive, slow manner. This art can get them to speed up and become much more active and vibrant. Bagua is also particularly valuable for helping people flow smoothly during periods of high, almost unbearable pressure and unpredictable situations. It provides a powerful antidote to the fast pace of change in modern life.

Tai chi tends to present its challenges in its meticulousness, requiring attention to many details. Those who reach a very high level in tai chi tend to like focusing on fine detail very deeply inside their being. Tai chi doesn't look as challenging as bagua because its complexities are not visible to the naked eye.

Tai chi is particularly valuable for someone who is overstressed, such as the classic type-A personality who could benefit from slowing down and becoming calmer. Letting go, relaxing and yielding in the many situations where there is no way to exert control can add to quality of life. Tai chi is the most popular stress-reduction program used by the successful business and professional classes in the booming economies of East Asia.

Tai chi is soft, round and feminine in approach. Tai chi is psychologically valuable for anyone who wants to successfully join together the yin elements of receptivity and sensitivity with the yang elements of strength and the capacity to accomplish goals.

However, because of the very yin or passive nature of tai chi, it can produce passive-aggressive individuals if the energy it generates goes to its negative aspect. In contrast, if the energy created from bagua goes to its very negative aspect, it tends to produce actively aggressive personalities.

Learning Curves

Many beginning tai chi students have problems with the coordination and sheer number of movements. Tai chi short forms are practiced by many more practitioners than long forms for two basic reasons. In a busy time-starved world, it takes less time to learn the movements of short forms and then fewer minutes to practice them.

Having taught more than 10,000 people tai chi, I have found that the physical coordination and memory required to learn and remember the large volume of movements of long forms are the main reasons why most people quit tai chi. Many who start don't stay with tai chi long enough to reap its plethora of health benefits or learn its meditation practices.

From this perspective, bagua has real advantages because there are fewer movements to learn. People with busy lives may find it much more doable, especially as beginners. You can choose to focus more on its health and meditative qualities and bypass many difficult physical coordination issues that are inherent in tai chi.

Space Requirements

Tai chi forms, particularly its long forms, take up a lot of practice space. You can't practice the long form in a small living room without running into a wall or some piece of furniture. You have to keep on stepping backward or sideways, which breaks the form's natural movement structures. Shorter forms can generally be practiced in smaller spaces.

When first learning bagua, you need even more room than tai chi. This is because you will need to walk in a fairly large circle as this is easier on your knees. Over time, however, the relative space requirements shift. As your skill in bagua grows, you can walk a smaller and smaller circle. When practicing bagua as meditation, you only need to perform the movements of the Single Palm Change. Once your circle gets smaller, you can practice in a room smaller than what even the shortest forms of tai chi require.

Improving Health

Neither bagua nor tai chi is intrinsically better or worse for improving health. Both can

- Balance and strengthen your chi
- Help to heal your internal organs
- Optimize the flow and circulation of all the fluids of your body, especially blood and interstitial fluid.

These are the healing capacities for which qigong is universally respected in Chinese medicine.

However, bagua and tai chi have their unique comparative advantages. Tai chi primarily heals through the yin nourishing principles of Chinese medicine while bagua heals through yang strengthening and tonifying principles.

If you are in good shape and you want to become super-healthy—as strong as humanly possible—bagua will help you accomplish this more easily than tai chi.

The low-impact nature of tai chi allows you to practice when you are injured or recovering from illness. As I did, you can use tai chi to help to heal yourself even straight out of the hospital. In general, if you are ill, in poor health or constitutionally weak, tai chi will help heal your body, and get your health and stamina back more easily and quickly. If you have fairly average overall health, but your major problem is stress that shreds your nervous system, then tai chi rather than bagua is best to help you slow down and calm your nervous system.

However, if your nervous system doesn't have the capacity to move fast enough to meet the demands of high-pressure work, then bagua might be more effective for you than tai chi.

Dealing with Health Problems

Bagua and tai chi are each suited to dealing with different kinds of health problems.[3] As a general rule, tai chi is better for diseases where nourishing the body's chi will help it heal. In Chinese medicine, this is classified as being yin deficient.

---

[3] If you have any medical or psychological problems, it is recommended that you consult your physician or healthcare provider to determine whether exercises, such as bagua and tai chi, are suitable for you. These practices are not meant to be used for diagnosis or treatment of specific conditions.

Bagua is better for diseases where the body's chi needs to be strengthened. In Chinese medicine, this is classified as tonifying the yang.

Tai chi is more effective at healing in cases where you need to balance your chi and build up extremely depleted chi. Severe diseases tend to cause this depletion. Bagua works better if the cause of your health problems is that the baseline strength of your chi is insufficient to spark powerful body regeneration.

If you have chronic fatigue syndrome, tai chi likely will be more helpful, especially if practiced in a very yin manner. In this case, your chi is not only depleted, but out of balance. Bagua might make you feel worse. However, when the more severe symptoms of chronic fatigue fade, bagua is more effective because it helps return your body to its previous full-operating capacity.

If you have carpal tunnel syndrome, bagua has an edge over tai chi because of the specialized ways it works the arms, hands and fingers.[4]

If you have low blood pressure, you would be much better off practicing bagua than tai chi. However, if you have very high blood pressure, tai chi may help you bring it down more effectively than bagua. In 1998, a study presented at the American Heart Association's Annual Conference on Cardiovascular Disease Epidemiology and Prevention by Deborah R. Young, PhD, assistant professor at the Johns Hopkins University School of Medicine in Baltimore, confirmed that tai chi lowered blood pressure for older adults.[5]

If you have back problems, rather than doing bagua, you should generally practice tai chi or qigong. However, if you have weak kidneys, but not a bad back, practicing bagua is best.

Bagua and tai chi address different emotional health issues. In many cases of low-grade depression, getting your internal systems moving considerably faster can pull you out of it. In this case, bagua would be more useful than tai chi, which might slow down your system. However, if the nature of your depression is combined with anger that frequently makes you flip out, then you would be better off practicing tai chi as it could cool your temper and calm you down.

---

[4] If you have repetitive strain injury (RSI) or other joint or back problems, be sure to consult your physician before taking up bagua or tai chi to make sure such exercises are appropriate for your specific condition.

[5] American Heart Association. "T'ai Chi Lowers Blood Pressure for Older Adults." *ScienceDaily* (March 20, 1998). Retrieved from *www.sciencedaily.com/releases/1998/03/980320075947.htm.*

Choreography and Spontaneity

Tai chi strongly emphasizes the choreography of its many movements. Although it has unique and specific chi techniques or principles for individual external movements, the basic program is distinctly choreographed. So the second move follows the first move, the third move follows the second move and so on. The core of a tai chi form is very much about having precise, deliberate movements that allow you to release your nervous system progressively and systematically. This sets the stage for the innate capacities of the mind and body to release all blockages and flourish.

Like tai chi, bagua also has choreography in the sense that it has specific movements. In bagua's martial art tradition, some of the movements are very similar to those practiced in tai chi long forms.

Unlike tai chi, however, bagua's changes of direction and progressions from one movement to the next are not predetermined. In Circle Walking, although move two follows movement one, it may not happen immediately.

Bagua's emphasis is less on performing precise external movements. Instead, the focus is on being able to change fluidly within any specific movement from one state into another. This is true for physical, energetic, emotional, mental and spiritual changes. The ability to spontaneously and smoothly change an external movement, such as changing direction and/or hand positions while Circle Walking, or an internal movement, such as shifting from one energetic state to another in one of your eight energy bodies, is at the core of bagua. It is the way you can completely shift your central nervous system and mind.

In tai chi, the specific ways the arms and legs coordinate with the turning of the waist is its main emphasis. Footwork and changing direction is the main emphasis in bagua's Circle Walking. Although the hand movements are coordinated with foot movements, that coordination is nowhere as critical in terms of precise choreography as it is in tai chi. As a general rule, bagua footwork is more complex and complete than that found in tai chi, and requires much more training.

Although both bagua and tai chi emphasize spontaneity in their martial sparring techniques, when it comes to solo practice, bagua has a much greater emphasis on spontaneity than tai chi. Tai chi places a much greater emphasis on regulated, rhythmic movement.

Circular and Spiral Movements Facilitate Fluidity

Bagua and tai chi are based upon seamless continuity and fluidity—first in your body, next your chi, then your mind and eventually your spirit.

Both arts are based on circular movement. Your body becomes a bit like a squid in the manner that you fold and articulate different parts of your torso, arms and legs. The body is trained until it seems boneless, so it can change and move in countless ways. Tai chi tends to do this in a circular manner, whereas bagua uses more obvious spiraling movement patterns.

Circles are two-dimensional while spirals are three-dimensional. Generally, most tai chi styles do not emphasize spiraling movement to the degree that bagua does, although the Chen style of tai chi comes close. Tai chi's overarching emphasis is on circular movement, which tends to be only in a single directional plane at any given moment.

Conversely, bagua's main focus is on spiraling movement, which can simultaneously involve multiple planes of movement at any given moment. Fluidity must always occur while three critical movement qualities are simultaneously present:

- Constant turning of the waist
- Bending (retraction) and stretching (extension) of the arms and legs toward and away from the torso
- Moving the limbs toward (inward) and away from the torso's centerline (outward) both forward, backward and sideways.

Fluidity must also derive from a very strong emphasis on total relaxation, softness or lack of rigidity within the body. In beginning practices, tai chi emphasizes softening the body. Bagua emphasizes twisting and internally strengthening the body until it becomes capable of relaxed fluid movement in any direction that the body's structure and anatomy safely allows.

Both bagua and Chen style tai chi also make undulating motions that are extremely rhythmic and include arm whipping actions.

Waist Movement and Footwork

Bagua and tai chi turn and reverse direction with waist turning. In tai chi, the main focal point is on waist movement with footwork as a subcategory. The feet are less emphasized because much of the time you are not moving your feet. Instead, you assume a position and shift your weight back and forth while turning your waist.

In bagua, the primary emphasis is on footwork. Waist turning is a subcategory of footwork. The first and foremost objective is to originate your motion in the feet rather than the waist. Your hand or waist never moves by itself. Instead, the movements are generated by your feet moving either in space or at least by changing pressures against the ground. At all practice levels, your feet must never stand still in one place for more than a fraction of a second.

As you turn or reverse direction in bagua and tai chi, it is extremely important to maintain your root at all times. This is true whatever the speed or direction of the movement and whether you are standing still or moving. The practitioner seeks to eliminate a bouncing, vertical up and down motion from one step to the next. The motion of your feet and the shifting of the weight should maintain a smooth continuum from one position to the next.

Hidden versus Obvious Power

Tai chi's power isn't easy to observe. It tends to be hidden right from the very beginning, which is consistent with tai chi's yin nature. Over time, as the student develops significant internal power, the specific goal of tai chi is to make it invisible—much like that of a stealth bomber. In Yang style tai chi, this is referred to as "steel wrapped in cotton." If people look at a tai chi practitioner they won't see how much internal power he or she has and will only feel it if the practitioner chooses to exhibit it. The exception is the Chen style of tai chi, whose explosive shaking and discharging movements make power quite noticeable.

Even in the earlier stages of practice, bagua's power is significantly more obvious, which is consistent with its yang nature. The sheer flow and speed make it obvious to any observer that power lies behind the movement. However, even if some overt power remains visible, as a bagua practitioner grows more proficient, more of the internal power becomes seamless and invisible. Eventually, it becomes impossible to figure out from where the practitioner's power is generated.

Working with the Chi of the Environment

For millennia, Taoists have worked with the five elemental energies: Metal, Water, Wood, Fire and Earth. All are present in the external environment. These elemental energies are brought into the practitioner's body and then in an opposite manner projected outward to affect what is in the external environment outside of the practitioner's physical body. Bagua and tai chi, especially in their more intact Taoist spiritual traditions, still practice this work.

At the level of internal energy work, bagua rather than tai chi practitioners have a much greater tendency to play with the energies of manifestation. They can develop a path for drawing energy from the environment into their bodies and minds, and then projecting that chi externally.

Most of the energetic work in tai chi is self-contained. However, you may move the energy out to the boundary of your etheric body, a distance of five to six feet or even ten feet away from your body. In tai chi, your chi is confined in a more defined space. In bagua, there is a tendency for the mind to roam greater distances and play with the energies of the environment around you in a much larger and more fluid way. The exception is at the much more advanced spiritual levels of tai chi: As meditation, one of its goals is to directly link the practitioner's body and mind with energies of the earth and heaven—reaching to the farthest galaxies.

At higher levels, especially in Taoist meditation practices, bagua tends toward activity, which reflects its emphasis on yang. Tai chi tends to be much more passive or yin. Tai chi is passive in the sense that it *follows* the flow or pressure of the air surrounding you. The way the chi flows inside your body that is influenced by the chi flowing in the air around you then causes, or at least significantly influences, your external movements. Bagua tends to be much more proactive in terms of initially creating chi flows inside your body to in turn create both external movements and chi flows in your etheric field. This further activates your internal chi flows and external movements.

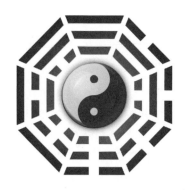

CHAPTER 8
Arts of Meditative Movement

As soon as you start to learn the basic movements of any genuine form of bagua or tai chi, you will experience a beginning aspect of their practice as meditation arts: meditative movement. Regardless of whether your interest is health, longevity, healing, martial arts or meditation, bagua and tai chi practice requires that you initially learn to move in a meditative manner—slowly, carefully, and with a relaxed focus and awareness. It requires you to develop capacities that are the foundation for almost any form of meditation, especially Taoist moving meditation. This includes the ability to recognize and apply progressively more subtle levels of your awareness, and focusing for extended periods on specific inner qualities with minimal distraction.

As your mind becomes stable and calm, you gain
- Constancy of purpose
- Feeling in all parts of your body
- Awareness of subtle layers within your body
- The ability to focus on specific inner qualities with minimal distraction for extended periods
- Relaxed awareness without which you would not be able to sustain the previous capacities for more than a few moments.

Bagua and tai chi open up, free and relax the nervous system and energy channels of your body. This creates healthy, strong and stable physical and etheric bodies, the latter of which is made up of the basic chi that runs your physical body (see pp. 28–30 on the eight energy bodies).

Stabilizing your mind and nervous system will help you more smoothly release energetic blockages and run all the higher energy bodies through your physical and etheric bodies. Creating an open, clear and awake mind that is capable of great elasticity is a fundamental practice in Taoism. It is how the principles of the *I Ching* are realized at the levels of the third, fourth, fifth and sixth energy bodies.

As you progress in learning bagua or tai chi, at no point is there a clear-cut dividing line between the results of bagua or tai chi for exercise or meditation; they are two sides of the same coin. You gain more calmness and clarity and progressively and systematically upgrade your overall health and wellness. Even beginners will recognize improvements and changes for the better.

Initially, your primary emphasis must be on developing vibrant health and energy. Proficiency in bagua or tai chi as qigong exercise provides the foundation necessary for learning Taoist or other meditation methods. This includes developing a relaxed, continuous and stable focus.

If you decide to become a more advanced Taoist meditation practitioner, your emphasis will gradually shift to learning ever more profound meditation methods. However, making your body healthier continues as a strong secondary focus of your practice. A healthy body and mind allow you to access powerful spiritual energies to resolve blockages using deeper Taoist meditation methods.

Developing the Foundation for Meditation

Bagua and tai chi practices are designed to strengthen and smooth your nervous system, which is necessary to acquire a calm, focused mind and healthy body. As you reduce and release stress, you also create more internal cohesion and with it whole-body awareness. This is a stepping stone to whole-mind awareness.

The conscious mind is only a small part of your whole mind. Most are aware of conscious thought. Relatively few are consciously aware of the subtle currents that flow through the unconscious or the even more subtle spiritual components that comprise the deepest layers of the human mind.

Stress Reduction

In the Taoist meditation tradition, stress reduction is a critical first step. Early stages of meditation are about teaching you how to relax and balance the energy flows inside your body. Stress destroys chi, leaving people unbalanced, erratic, unfocused and sometimes deranged. Stress breaks down the body and mind.

Once you can manage the stresses of daily life, the subject of the complete spiritual unfolding of the human soul can be addressed. If people cannot manage the simple day-to-day stresses of life, the idea that they can become spiritually evolved is little more than wishful thinking.

Stress Spikes Your Nervous System

During times of stress, the nerves go from having an ideally balanced, even, coordinated flow to having irregular and uneven spikes. The mind either becomes agitated and frenetic (or even manic), or subdued and depressive. When that occurs, the body may produce adrenaline and other destructive hormones as a defense mechanism. The process can become habitual as a result of repeated stressful catalysts, creating a negative feedback loop.

Bagua's method of regularizing these spikes is to Walk the Circle while holding one hand in front of your eyes and continuously looking at your index finger (the upper body palm posture). While doing this simple physical act, you keep your

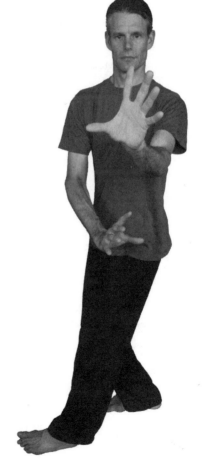

Photo by Bill Walters

Bagua Single Palm Change Posture.

focus either on your finger or the rhythm of your walking. In time this smoothes and steadies the nerves.

If your nervous system spikes or your mind drifts, the weight of your arm and your need to stay walking your circle will help bring you back into focus. A seesaw effect is thus induced between constantly losing and regaining your focus. In order for you to accomplish the tasks of staying on your circle and watching your finger, through repetition your mind will eventually find a way to relax and open up.

However, the only way your mind can truly open is by having the signals in your nervous system become steady. So you continue Walking the Circle. The focus of the mind is particularly strengthened as you change direction or alter your speed.

Tai chi's approach to smoothing the spikes of the nervous system is to establish steady, rhythmical patterns of movement that progressively relax and soothe it. Your mind is trained to stay focused on performing the myriad details that are required by each movement. If your mind jumps or drifts, or your nervous system spikes, you'll be thrown off the sequence of movements. Then you'll realize you need to refocus and get back on track.

As bagua and tai chi strengthen the nervous system, you will notice a reduction in the frequency of instances when your nerves become overstimulated. This is because your nervous system is growing stronger and more stable. Avoiding over-stimulation allows your mind to remain more quiet, calm and focused.

Stress Decreases Mental Agility

A major problem with stress is that the mind loses its ability to be nimble and agile, so you are more inflexible and easily fixate on one idea or another. This is especially true for expectations or desires. When suddenly confronted with upheaval, the emotions can take over and freeze your ability to act. That is why many stress management programs are geared toward helping people learn to accept situations for what they are and find a way out of their self-imposed mental boxes. They aim to teach people how to respond appropriately to the needs of the moment rather than getting stuck in endlessly churning mental loops.

Bagua and tai chi do the same. They are great stress management tools for helping you stay in the moment and avoid spacing out.

When you practice bagua or tai chi you must constantly change your physical orientation. You adjust where your eyes look and your head faces, moving from place to place in a very steady way. You are meant to do this without getting stuck in the middle of a movement. If you find yourself physically stuck, or more importantly, emotionally or mentally stuck, your movements will immediately become rigid and you may even forget what you are doing. At this point, you try to quickly get back on track; smoothing your mind and emotions so that your physical movements can once again become continuous. Over time, your focus will grow and stabilize, and your emotions and mental churnings become less predisposed to roller-coaster rides.

In the process of constantly smoothing out the physical and energetic movements within your bagua or tai chi, you train your mind to become more flexible. Your mind has no choice but to constantly adapt to physically transiting between where it was and where it will be. Eventually, you give up some of the attachments associated with inflexibility, such as: "This shouldn't be happening"; "This can't be happening" or "Something else should be happening." Practicing the movements gradually trains your mind to let go of places where you habitually get stuck, thereby creating a more agile mind.

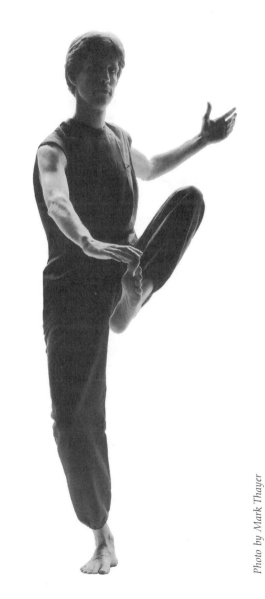

Photo by Mark Thayer

The Repulse Monkey posture from the Wu style tai chi long form, a movement that is challenging in terms of physical balance.

THE CHI OF WANG SHU JIN: THE BUDDHA BELLY

Although Wang Shu Jing usually didn't like to kick or lift his legs up very much, his arms could move like lightning. However, it was what he gave off with his constant turning and twisting that really gave me a sense of what it meant to develop a chi belly. The Chinese and Japanese call the energy point in this area the *lower tantien* or *hara*, respectively. Both cultures regard the lower tantien as the real center of the physical body's chi.

The power of Wang's Buddha belly personified for me how everything in bagua comes out of the lower tantien and returns into it. I could feel his chi swirling around my body and giving me what amounted to a contact high—just by being in his vicinity.

Wang could move the inside of his physical body in a very condensed manner, as if it were made of dense rubber accompanied by a very expansive chi. He had an immense energy field around him that was generated from the energy field inside his body.

Practicing outdoors in the winter in Taiwan, Wang would put his very fleshy hand out to students so they could grab it and warm up their hands. After a while, you realized that Wang could make his hand hot simply by applying chi with his intent. After experiencing this a few times, he suggested that we not wear gloves around him while practicing in order to bring out our chi.

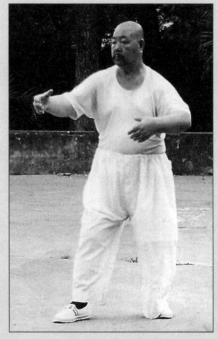

Photo by author

Wang gave me a sense of movement and chi that was very real and tangible. By hanging around there was an unambiguous sense that things were moving both inside your own body and in his—below the skin right into the body's core. Along with that, he absolutely brought home that bagua movement could make a person physically powerful with immense control and very vibrant energy.

Developing a Strong Center

Bagua and tai chi also help you develop a sense of internal cohesion and whole-body awareness, physically and mentally. In order to coordinate and align all moving parts—hands, feet, waist and twisting motions—you must have a strong center.

Fulfilling the physical requirements of the Single Palm Change or a tai chi form requires you to move your body as a connected whole rather than a series of loosely connected or uneven jerky parts. Your mind must also be coherent: constant, stable and focused. In order to smoothly navigate the continuously changing movements, bagua and tai chi naturally stimulate the development of a strong, psychological center within you. Over time, it fuses into the physical and energetic center of the lower tantien (see Appendix C).

Many people have the sense that they're one kind of person in one situation and a different person in another. They do not have an overriding sense of continuity between the moments of their life because there is minimal constancy or cohesion of mind.

Bagua, with its constant Circle Walking and changes of direction, or tai chi, with its constant waist turning and shifts from one movement to another, give you a process that accustoms the mind to making changes yet remaining internally cohesive. You don't accomplish this by only thinking and philosophizing about it. You must learn how to *do* it. By undergoing physical training with continuously repeating movements, in time your mind progressively unifies and moves through the changes without instigating a stress response.

You try not to fixate on a single idea of what being centered means. Your sense of cohesion and center being more amorphous will more smoothly link and hold everything together within you. Then, no matter what you're going through, you can handle it without effort or strain.

Foster Whole-body Awareness

The complex nature of bagua and tai chi's movements eventually leads to a sense of whole-body connectedness or awareness. At first, you mentally think of specific movements—keeping a hand at a certain height, changing positions, moving your foot or hip and a myriad of other physical details. Because you have to think about the movements, a fusing of the body and mind occurs. Combined with attention to the sixteen neigong components, your ability to feel and be aware of your entire body naturally develops. In order to accomplish so many things at once, your mind must relax and remain open to encompass effortless multitasking.

Without developing some degree of internal mental cohesion, whole-body awareness is impossible to attain. From the other side of the coin, training to achieve whole-body awareness must, of necessity, increase your internal cohesion. These qualities are necessary to practice the beginning stages of Taoist meditation.

Sinking Your Chi to Sink Your Mind

At the simplest level, meditation is about settling the mind so it is capable of deep and powerful focus. Bagua and tai chi, like Zen Buddhism, accomplish this by teaching you to sink your body's chi into the lower tantien. You draw your mind's awareness inward and downward where eventually—with much personal refinement—it becomes stable and awakens the body's central channel of energy.

Developing a Relaxed Body and Mind

Bagua and tai chi's foundational meditation practices are designed to develop a mind that is attentive, focused, relaxed, balanced and stable, which creates a relaxed body. Although it is possible to have a relaxed mind inside a tense body, it is definitely easier and more sustainable to relax the mind within a relaxed body.

Bagua and tai chi use strategies for developing an integrated body and mind.

Tai chi focuses on the space inside your body. Within regular, rhythmical, slow movements that naturally relax your body, your mind must concentrate on the many movements, chi flows and physical details of the form. The only way your mind can pull this off is by relaxing and opening. This is a first step in using meditation methods to tap into the tai chi space of emptiness that is beyond opposites.

Developing relaxed concentration skills requires you to focus on more than the constant and regular body changes from yin to yang to yin. These include
  • Opening and closing
  • Bending and stretching
  • Twisting in and out
  • Inhaling and exhaling.

You must also focus on the empty space in between the yin and yang when you make the changeovers. Tai chi is about smoothly alternating your moves with a very steady rhythm.

In bagua, you intensely focus your attention internally and externally while continuously changing direction and speed. The aim is to physically and mentally move through change without resistance. This is only possible through relaxation.

Bagua focuses on what is happening physically and energetically as you make each change and shift between yin and yang, often in the blink of an eye. Internally and smoothly moving through change, regardless of how slow, sudden or unpredictable, is bagua's specialty.

The Joys of Spiritual Greed

All genuine Eastern practices—including martial, healing and meditative arts—contain a very simple idea: Don't be in a rush to go to the next step. Weak foundations easily create crumbling buildings and you don't build a house from the third story down.

Because we live in an acquisitive society that emotionally rewards people for the amount of their possessions—whether material or intellectual—many students do not realize that body/mind/spirit skills require a very different approach.

Skills in the Eastern arts are carefully and progressively crafted. End goals involve building and balancing chi and moving toward spirituality, so you can't skip the basics. In the West, many students of chi practices like to collect movements, sets or energy arts the way a child would marbles. However, in China the focus is not on how many marbles you have, but how well you understand and can use them.

The race to develop and flaunt superior abilities, to pile up skill upon skill, and to aggressively compete in their acquisition are forms of spiritual greed. They are the antithesis of the Taoist ideals of balance and compassion.

Greed for knowledge of chi drives many to attempt advancing to step three before they have learned steps one or two. You must put away whatever fantasy you might have about the rewards of jumping ahead before you're ready. Take the time necessary for learning all the nuances of each new step before moving forward.

THE CHI OF HUNG I HSIANG: AN UNDULATING SNAKE

Six years after I met Wang Shu Jin, I encountered Hung I Hsiang. He was my next major bagua teacher who lived in Taipei, Taiwan. At that time, Hung taught very little Circle Walking. Rather he taught a kind of linear bagua, and a type of hsing-i, which was infused from beginning to end with the principles and movement style of bagua.

Hung was another teacher who had a large girth. Yet he had a quality that was extremely noticeable from the perspective of moving energy. The inside of Hung's body was like a massive, coiling undulating snake or amoeba. His movements had a total rubberlike quality, which could freely shift from here to there and back again. It was always coming out of a completely stable core as though he had no bones anywhere in his body. Hung's reflexes were amazingly quick and light, with his chi manifesting itself as an ability to move with incredibly dramatic and rapidly shifting micro-movements.

It was obvious that he had refined and developed the micro-physical movements of his hands, as well as the aliveness of his belly and tantien. When he touched someone using a martial art technique, I could feel tiny little waves throughout his system and immense micro-control of everything inside his abdomen, internal organs, muscles and joints. He demonstrated masterful adaptations of many of the sixteen neigong components.

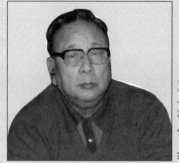

Photo by H. L. Lei

Without a Beginning, There Is No End

Practicing the preparatory work and not reflexively skipping ahead is required to realistically obtain the benefits of the next, more advanced technique. Without taking the time to lay a strong foundation, any advanced technique you may perform to some degree will lack the capacity to bring forth its true potential. An aspiring guitarist cannot skip straight ahead to wonderful riffs without first taking the time to master basic chords.

THE CHI OF LIU HUNG CHIEH:
THE ELASTICITY OF A RUBBER BAND

When I met my teacher Liu in his late seventies, he was so skinny that I could easily put my fingers around his thigh. He was about 5'2" and probably weighed less than 110 pounds. A quality you couldn't help but notice was the extreme looseness of his shoulders.

He had lived through China's Communist Revolution, Great Leap Forward and Cultural Revolution without eating much food for some thirty to forty years. It wasn't that he didn't want to; he just had little access to any food.

Liu could move exceedingly smoothly and well for a person of any age, let alone someone fairly old who, by his early seventies, had severely damaged his hip sockets from frostbite.

The most noticeable quality about his body was that it was like a massive rubber band. His body went beyond being boneless; it was as though he was elastic.

This was very freaky because the guy was also inhumanly powerful. At that time, I was a very big, strong man. Yet in terms of physical power, Liu could control me as though I were a baby.

What was highly unusual was that along with his ability to generate immense power—in both bagua and tai chi—he emitted a complete sense of his body being absolutely quiet and at peace with itself. I've never observed this quality in anybody before or since.

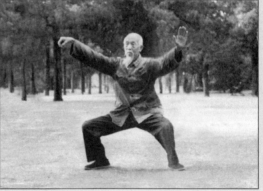

Photo by author

Malcolm Gladwell's best-selling book, *Outliers,*[1] analyzes people who have excelled well beyond the norm. One of his essential points is that virtually no one achieves great success and mastery without spending 10,000 hours or about ten years practicing. Gladwell points out that prodigies and overnight successes are extremely rare.

---

[1] Little Brown and Company, 2008.

My experience learning bagua, tai chi and meditation is consistent with his findings. When describing qualifications, genuine tai chi masters commonly advised: It takes ten years of diligent effort before you are ready to leave the courtyard and walk the land.

As you move into more advanced practices, the lessons become progressively more difficult and subtle. Typically, new steps that might appear to have only minor differences actually take time to master and can make a huge difference to your overall progress. This applies not only to improving steps you have already learned, but also to when you integrate new skills later on. The subtleties determine how much value you can reap from your practice.

Regardless of the speed of your natural learning curve, an interesting point occurs as you keep layering more techniques on top of another: There is no way to predict which layer will take you longest to successfully make solid and comfortable. Nor can you predict when adding a layer too fast might wind up crumbling everything below it, setting you back to zero.

Don't rush yourself. Enjoy the process of letting go of that which stands in your way.

Building a solid foundation is an absolutely necessary precursor to reaping the fruits of spiritual knowledge. Spiritual greed in any form will not only take away the joy in learning, but will defeat your ability to learn in the first place and prevent genuine satisfaction.

The Wonderful Accident

For the average bagua or tai chi practitioner interested in exercise, the basic meditation practices the arts contain will serve primarily as a means to manage stress and calm an anxiety-driven mind. Yet with practice almost everyone will experience the odd moment when they catch a glimpse of their spiritual essence. They are suddenly left within themselves. A residue of inner peace may remain that is more profound than most people experience in a lifetime. In Taoism this is what is called the "wonderful accident." Such experiences often inspire people to commit to engage in the more advanced practices of Taoist meditation.

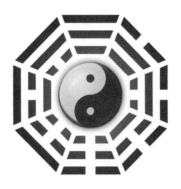

CHAPTER 9
Profound Methods
of Taoist Meditation

If at some point you have the opportunity to practice bagua and tai chi in a genuine Taoist meditation tradition, then you will go beyond movements that help you become healthier and calm your mind. You will engage in a profound spiritual path.

Bagua is the primary Taoist moving meditation art of the *I Ching*. Nevertheless, the foundations of tai chi serve similar functions based on the methodologies of the *I Ching*. These include working with the eight energy bodies while laying the foundation for higher levels of meditation. At these advanced stages, bagua and tai chi have unique ways of climbing the mountain to reach its summit.

As you progress through the stages of Taoist moving meditation, bagua and tai chi as exercise have more powerful effects. Greater energy and health penetrate right into the marrow of your bones.

Old age, illness or injury—the inherent limitations of having a physical body—will eventually catch up with all of us. However, the farther along the Taoist exercise-meditation continuum you travel, the more capacity you have for managing and overcoming limitations as you age. This is true of physical, emotional and mental setbacks. The real gifts of bagua and tai chi as exquisite exercise and profound meditation are a significantly more balanced and joyful life.

Stages of Taoist Meditation

Committing to the path of Taoist or any serious form of meditation is much like attending a religious school for many years. In the Taoist tradition, spirituality does not come like a bolt of lightning from the sky or simply because you want it. You learn by deeply exploring your innermost internal landscape. The potential for spirituality lies within all of us, although realization for most ordinary mortals involves a long and sustained effort.

The advanced practices of Taoist meditation take you through three distinct stages that progressively penetrate deeper inside yourself. These stages, of necessity, must be done in the following sequence. After you have more or less fully completed one stage, then you are ideally primed to embark on the next.

1. **Become a fully mature human being** who is essentially free of inner conflicts and inner demons. In this stage, you completely release all the small and large conditionings, tensions and blockages that bind and prevent your soul from reaching its full spiritual potential.
2. **Reach inner stillness.** Taoist meditation practice will take you to a place deep inside you that is absolutely still, permanent and stable. This place does not waiver, whether you are quietly sitting or doing fifty things at once.
3. **Transform the body, mind and spirit** through internal alchemy until you merge with the Tao.

In all three stages, you gradually open, clear and integrate the eight energy bodies within you as you progress from jing-chi-shen-wu-Tao or body-energy-spirit-emptiness-Tao.

Bagua and tai chi practices equally emphasize emotional and mental transformation. However, the specific ways and techniques by which they access the depths of human consciousness and take you through the complete journey to the Tao are different, just as two dishes might use the same raw ingredients yet each have a unique flavor.

The three stages of Taoist meditation can only be learned from a living Taoist master and, depending on the school, may be taught through sitting, standing, moving, lying down or interactive practices. As with any authentic tradition, within Taoism there are many schools and subdivisions. Finding a teacher adept in the depth of these practices is of the utmost importance as discussed in Chapter 10.

The Road to Maturity and Inner Stillness

In the Taoist meditation tradition, the road to maturity and inner stillness has three abiding principles.

The Past Is Not Your Future

Whatever is within the deeper recesses of your psyche is not set in stone. If something tears you apart inside, know that it is possible to release all your internal conversations about perceived hurts, and any resentment or feelings of "they made me do it" or "they did it to me."

You can release all the internal limitations your past has imposed upon you, particularly those you've used to create your self-identity and that dictate, at the depths of your unconscious, how you should think and act.

You Have the Power

You have the power to take responsibility for your life. This may not necessarily mean being responsible for the trials and tribulations inevitable in living, but how you interpret, respond to and handle them. You can free your spirit from taking on unnecessary internal burdens as you travel the road of internal freedom.

You Are More than Your Personality

Most people think, "I am my personality." The more you free yourself from being fixated on either the yin or yang of your personality—the "this" and the "that" of any situation—the more easily you will find the place that allows you to balance both sides simultaneously. Taoists call this the "tai chi space."

Becoming Mature

Mature individuals can relax and function well amid life's imperfections. They do not need acknowledgment for their accomplishments. They do not pass judgment on others. Maturity practices are about moving you toward personal freedom from conditioned emotions and thought patterns. As long as you possess internal demons that keep you spinning like a hamster on its wheel you cannot be natural. Your innermost soul must relax and let go of conditionings, which can take many years.

Reaching maturity and inner stillness involves many progressive phases:

- Developing the ability to focus your mind until you can maintain concentration on subtle qualities beyond mundane tasks. If you cannot keep your mind focused steadily on genuine spiritual matters, interest in them too easily becomes a series of fleeting, feel-good, unpleasant or simply entertaining experiences.
- Exploring the meaning of morality.
- Focusing your inner awareness for exceptionally long periods on subtle energetic, mental or psychic phenomena that may initially seem invisible or extremely opaque.
- Externally focusing on an activity, yet remaining internally calm.
- Smoothing and unblocking energy channels.
- Releasing, letting go of and resolving your inner demons, traumas and personal faults.
- Remaining calm, so that you are capable of handling multiple, very intense whirlwinds of life without becoming ruffled.
- Activating your spiritual potential for higher levels of awareness within your internal organs and glands.
- Using the esoteric Five Elements (Metal, Water, Wood, Fire and Earth) that underlie the manifestation of matter and events.
- Transcending emotional and psychic negativity that limits your capacity for balance and compassion.
- Truly being in the present moment and living your life from a timeless place beyond past, present and future.
- Developing a mind and spirit that rests in inner stillness, thus gaining the ability to penetrate to the essence of matters and see beyond appearances to their root.

Developing Spiritual Morality

You must fully explore the meaning of spiritual morality or *Tao De*—the morals or virtues of the Tao—to achieve inner stillness. You must engage in deep self-exploration to understand how morality creates your inner psychic and emotional environment. You must also recognize and deal with a host of external and internal causes and effects, often called "karma" in the West.

Questions naturally arise that demand soul-searching answers: What is virtue? Why be moral? How should morality be expressed? What place should human emotions, in terms of morality, have in the grand scheme? Should emotions or thoughts be moderated or thrown about with a damn-the-consequences attitude? What is the essential nature of morality, love, compassion, wisdom, spontaneity and generosity? If morality is withheld, how does it shred the fabric of your soul and society in general?

Going through this process will give you a sound footing in your inner world. It cuts the legs off much potential hypocrisy and forestalls needless rebellions that would otherwise drain energy and create problems for delving deeper into spiritual discovery.

If morality is omitted from the process, the danger exists that you might focus purely on gaining power. Lacking morality often results in making insecurities and spiritual defects even larger, which decreases the potential for transcending them.

Developing Internal Energy

The science of how energy flows in humans is neigong (see Chapter 2, pp. 12–14). It is the root from which all the Taoist qigong systems in China have obtained some or most of their technical information and potential capacities. It is also the root of the essential chi work of the internal martial arts (bagua, tai chi and hsing-i),[1] Taoist meditation, and Chinese medicine's qigong therapies and bodywork systems.

Learning bagua and tai chi commonly begins with learning basic movement forms. Bagua includes Circle Walking and/or the Single Palm Change. Tai chi has short or long form styles. Over time, neigong components are incorporated into

---

[1] The internal martial arts are also called *nei jia chuan*, or *neijiaquan*, which means "the family of martial arts based on neigong."

the movements at increasingly sophisticated levels with the goal of progressively opening up all the energy channels of the body, mind and spirit.

What makes learning these components unique to energetic practices is that they are learned as a circular process. On your first pass through a particular component, you may only learn its most basic elements. Then, on the next pass, you might move on to deeper aspects that you again incorporate into your physical movements. You return over and over again to specific neigong components to flesh out their more refined and powerful aspects and applications within the movements. The sequence of learning the sixteen components is not cast in stone, although many people find that learning the breathing and alignment components early on to be particularly useful for health and relaxation.

THE FRANTZIS ENERGY ARTS SYSTEM

Some of the essential physical and energetic components of qigong and neigong are taught as separate programs in the Frantzis Energy Arts® System. Each program focuses on specific health benefits and aspects of neigong. As the techniques of each program are learned, students integrate them and incorporate them into other practices, such as bagua, tai chi or sitting meditation.

The program includes: Longevity Breathing®; Dragon and Tiger Medical Qigong; Opening the Energy Gates of Your Body™ Qigong; Marriage of Heaven and Earth™ Qigong; Bend the Bow™ Spinal Qigong; Spiraling Energy Body™ Qigong; Gods Playing in the Clouds™ Qigong; and Taoist Longevity Yoga™.

Each qigong set was developed to help students focus on particular neigong components. For example, foundational alignments are taught in Opening the Energy Gates, and techniques for openings and closing are taught in the Marriage of Heaven and Earth.

Taking these programs before or at the same time as studying bagua or tai chi will accelerate your training in specific neigong components and help you incorporate them successfully into your practice. Each program builds and supports the next in a circular manner, enabling most students to start anywhere on the circle.

The sophistication of neigong is experienced by practitioners as progressive and systematic improvements in health and the energetic and spiritual capacities of the mind, body and spirit. This ever-deepening sophistication is what allows bagua and tai chi to become exquisite exercises and profound meditation vehicles for Taoist spiritual practices.

The talent and knowledge of your individual instructor, your own talent and the discipline you apply to your practice are the three factors that determine how and when you progress.

Bagua and tai chi are derived from neigong/qigong traditions of Taoist medita-tion. Qigong is the relatively modern term used for the term neigong that has been used for thousands of years. The term *gong* means "work." So *neigong* means the "work of internal chi development." *Qigong* means "working with chi" and in the current era this is considered a branch of Traditional Chinese Medicine.

Physical Layers of the Body and the Eight Energy Bodies

The highest goal of Taoist meditation is to become consciously aware of all eight energy bodies (see pp. 28–30) and clear and connect them all into one unified whole. This is the process of freeing the deepest recesses of your being. It goes far beyond mere physical and mental relaxation or improving health and peace of mind. Rather, it is relaxing into your soul or your very being. It's about finding the place of spirit and emptiness that is the Tao—universal consciousness itself.

As a general principle, you gradually progress from beginning with opening, releasing, freeing and enlivening the first two energy bodies (physical and etheric). You start with bagua or tai chi as qigong exercises, and then apply the same process for the remaining energy bodies. Although this is not strictly a linear process—from lower to higher frequency energy bodies—it is the general direction for deepening your practice.

Just as each energy body extends farther out into space than the previous one, each body individually resonates with progressively deeper layers inside your physical body. Each layer, which is between the skin and the body's innermost core, directly corresponds and relates to one of the first seven energy bodies. The deeper the layer, the more refined and the higher the frequency it resonates.

The eighth body of the Tao is beyond any physical resonance. The body of the Tao encompasses the entirety of all and everything.

For example, under the skin there is a layer of energy between the skin and the beginning of muscle, called *wei chi* in Chinese medicine. It resonates with the energies of your physical body and your second or etheric body. A deeper layer that contains the ligaments resonates with the energies of your third or emotional body.

Clearing blockages in each energy body involves applying the sixteen neigong components at ever-greater levels of sophistication. As you clear a blockage at one energetic level, the physical structure to which it is attached becomes healthier, stronger and more vibrant. This prepares you to be able to go deeper in your body and to take on deeper and more profound blockages.

The deeper that you are able to move into your body, the healthier and more vital it becomes. So as you clear blockages in ever more refined levels of your being, the exercise value of your bagua or tai chi continuously grows.

Five Energetic Practice Elements

There are five particularly important elements in the practice of bagua and tai chi as arts of developing chi for health or meditation. As all five come into play, in an aggregate, synergistic fashion they cause all the fluids of the body to circulate evenly and powerfully, including the blood and interstitial fluids between the cells.

1. Spiraling Energy

You want to develop a spiraling or twisting energy that involves all parts of the body including: the abdominal cavity, internal organs, bone marrow, tendons, ligaments, muscles and the deepest layers of fasciae. Sometimes the external twisting actions are obvious. Others occur so deeply within the body as to give minimal visual clues to those not thoroughly trained to specifically recognize them.

2. Six Combinations of the Body

Physically, a focus on the six combinations of the body *(liu he)*, refers to the three external pairs of combinations: the elbow with the knee; the hand with the foot;

and the shoulder with the hip. Each coordinates with the other through the center core of the body.

The three internal combinations—intention, energy and consciousness—must coordinate with one another as well as with the three external combinations of the physical body.

The object is to make the whole physical body, chi and mind move like one totally integrated cell without disconnected moving parts. Two of the most important phrases in tai chi illustrate this point perfectly: "From posture to posture the internal power remains unbroken," and "When one part moves, all parts move; when one part stops, all parts stop."

3. Body Systems Connected to the Spine

You want your movements to incorporate all the body systems connected to the spine. This process maximizes the strength and flexibility of the spinal column, helps to heal spinal injuries and develops the central nervous system's sensitivity, strength and stamina. Bagua and tai chi move the vertebrae of the spine continuously, powerfully pumping cerebrospinal fluid through the system.

4. Opening and Closing

You want to develop opening and closing in the joints and cavities of the body, including the expansion and compression of the synovial fluid within the joints. The openings and closings help free up the body's energy flows.

5. Energy Channels of the Body

An essential goal is to open the major energy channels of the body, and there are a lot of them. The most important three are the central, left and right channels (see Appendix C).

Other important energy channels include the body's yin and yang acupuncture meridians. Yin meridians run along the inside of the arms and legs and along the front of the body. The yang meridians run along the outside of the legs, along the back and on the outside of the arms.

There are also the acupuncture meridians that circle your body in the manner of connective belts (*jing luo*). Other important meridians include what are referred to as the eight special or extraordinary meridians. All these channels are opened and joined through the moving practices of bagua and tai chi.

Stirring Chi

When you move beyond the basic meditation methods of bagua and tai chi into their more profound spiritual levels, you will most likely alternate your moving meditation practices with standing, sitting, lying down or interactive modes, including sexual ones. For example, if you practice bagua or tai chi as martial arts, you may find that when participating in such interactive modes as sparring, Push Hands or Rou Shou, you will want to alternate your practice with standing, sitting or lying down methods of meditation.

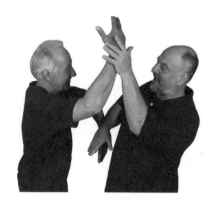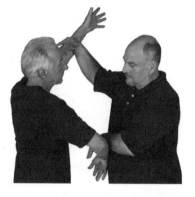

Photos by Bill Walters

Push Hands is the middle ground between tai chi solo form work and sparring. Here the author is teaching a student *Rou Shou* or Soft Hands, bagua's bridge from solo practice to fighting.

Bagua and tai chi's moving practices can stir up and activate dormant energies. They may affect structures and energetic flows deep inside the body that resonate with the fourth through seventh energy bodies (mental, psychic, karmic or causal and essence or body of individuality). While practicing movements, deeply bound energies can be released which otherwise would remain dormant.

In the most advanced practices, these energies consist of what the Taoists call our inner ghosts or demons—old emotional, mental or other patterns that commonly stay locked deep below the surface until their "button" is pushed. These can be released especially during practice of sparring or Push Hands, which can unleash dormant emotions of fear or aggression.[2]

Movement to Stillness and Stillness to Movement

Once these dormant energies are activated, standing, sitting or lying down meditation methods are combined with advanced neigong techniques to resolve and clear out whatever came up from the movements in a concentrated manner. These processes will eventually open up all the body's energy channels, 4,000 to 5,000 of which are functionally useful.

Circle Walking makes your "internal content" rise out of the depths so you can then more fully resolve blockages in that content while sitting. Eventually, the two practice methods merge. Sitting practice gives you the experience of resolving what comes up. Classically, you then take that experience back into your Circle Walking where it continues to drive you deeper into what needs to be transformed or resolved.

This alternation between methods can more rapidly bring about resolutions than just sitting or moving could do alone. In this way, sitting and Circle Walking reinforce each other—they are not separate practices. Each has the ability to uncover the blockages as well as the techniques to release them. Moving and sitting practices flow into and energize each other.

Applying Intent and Opening the Heart-Mind

The Heart-Mind is an important concept in Taoism and Buddhism. To understand the Heart-Mind in bagua and tai chi, you must first understand the nature of intent.

There are two levels of intent in everything you do in Taoism and Taoist chi work. The first is ordinary intent. The second level of intent is the place from which intent arises originally. That is, the place where intent is born. It could be said that this intent is beyond birth and death.

---

[2] Sparring practices, such as Push Hands, should only be practiced by those lacking serious psychological problems unless cleared by their healthcare practitioner.

Any level of intent has both a yin and yang component. If you want to walk across the street, that's a yang action because you have to do something. If you want something to come toward you, that's a yin form of intent.

But then there's the question of where the intent comes from to begin with: Where do all your thoughts come from? Where do all your emotions come from? Where is the birthing room of yin and yang?

As discussed in Chapter 2, classic Chinese philosophy says that in the beginning there was the undifferentiated void called wu chi (wu ji). Wu chi held within itself all possibilities, but was beyond needing to ever take form. However, in order for creation to come into existence, there needed to be a creative force. This force was called tai chi (taiji).

Tai chi gives birth to yin and yang. Tai chi is neutral. It can be either yin or yang, neither yin nor yang, or both. It has no qualities of its own, but its non-dual or non-differentiated quality allows any yin and yang to take form. It is a level of emptiness that produces manifestation.

So where does any thought, any emotion, any phenomena come from? If you have a psychic perception, where does it come from? If a thought comes into your mind, or an emotion comes into your body, from where does it originate? The thought itself, the emotion itself, the psychic perception itself, or even the way karma occurs itself always has a yin or a yang quality. It could be more yin and less yang or more yang and less yin, but one or both are always involved. You can break anything down in this way, from the tiniest things that exist at the quantum level to the biggest things in the universe.

The subconscious—a modality of thought—is still yin and yang. The place in the subconscious from where it is born is the Heart-Mind. It is not the subconscious itself, but rather the place that gives birth to the subconscious.

On a human level, intent is ordinary, but there is also another level: the Heart-Mind. Sometimes Taoists use the word *shen* (spirit). Buddhists always refer to the Heart-Mind, Taoists sometimes use the term Heart-Mind and sometimes use *shen*, but the fact is that they're interchangeable.

How do you reach the Heart-Mind? What is the method? Lao Tse's 2,500-year-old tradition of ice to water, water to inner space is Inner Dissolving. When you go from ice to water that's a yin-yang relationship; tension to relaxation is a yin-yang relationship.

If you want to go to the place where these energies originate, you effectively will move through two levels. On the level of human perception, to arrive at relaxation (or water) you will move through the subconscious whether you realize it or not. This process involves the transparency of recognizing the deeper implications of what's involved with a specific yin and yang. It's about becoming aware of the subtle nuances associated with that yin and yang, which, unless you have training, are not normally obvious. If you go one step farther into what really allows the subconscious to generate yin and yang, then you arrive at the Heart-Mind. This is what can be called spirit.

Some might consider the Heart-Mind to be the subconscious, but this is not a very accurate definition. However, given the fact that the West uses the conscious and subconscious dichotomy, it might help you understand the concept. Heart-Mind has no qualities, or you could say it has every quality. It's not yin and yang, or you could say that it has every possible yin and yang that could ever exist.

This place is then where you start the ice to water, water to inner space process (Inner Dissolving). The process of going to inner space is the process of going to emptiness. Emptiness only arises once the Heart-Mind is activated to a strong enough degree. How strong is the emptiness? To what degree is there emptiness? When you look at emptiness very closely, then you find that there are relative stages of emptiness and with recognizable qualities. The point is that each one of those stages comes from the Heart-Mind.

In the Western frame of thought, there are only two things: the conscious mind and the unconscious mind. In Eastern thought, there is a very distinct continuum that goes from gross yin-yang to subtle yin-yang to that which is beyond yin-yang. The subtlety is from where the subconscious comes. There's obvious intent and then there's the Heart-Mind from which intent ultimately arises. Awakening and engaging the Heart-Mind ultimately is a keystone of all higher level qigong and Taoist meditation.

When first learning qigong, you might have the intent for your chi to move. However, this is not the same as becoming directly aware of the chi itself, where it's a felt, living quality. It's not that you have only the idea, the imagination or the ability to think about chi, but that you actually feel and experience it. It's the difference between the idea of eating and actually eating—having the juices in your mouth and tasting the food. The idea will produce some facsimile of the real thing and you might go so far as to salivate. When the real deal is present, the taste and sustenance of the food is either there or it's not. There's little thought involved.

Similarly, in order to actually feel chi directly, you have to go through the Heart-Mind. You must have a direct experience of moving chi in the body, which requires that the Heart-Mind is open—even if only to the tiniest degree.

All qigong and meditation starts at the level of intent and arrives at the Heart-Mind.

Take the idea of Inner Dissolving. You want a release, you have the intent for a release, but then it goes past a certain point where you start awakening the Heart-Mind. It sits there with the willingness for something to happen, but then it shifts into something that becomes very real. This is where Lao Tse's Water tradition and the Fire traditions part company. Many of the Fire methods are very strongly based only upon ordinary intent.

To enter the real world of qigong, you have to access the Heart-Mind. At the level of intent, only a small percentage of your being is involved. The degree to which you attach the Heart-Mind—surface-level or deep involvement—is the degree to which your being is involved. If you want to awaken the latent parts of the brain, it can only be done after the Heart-Mind is functioning really well.

Whether you're using only intent or you're accessing the Heart-Mind, normally you'll be doing the same actions or techniques. The only difference is that once you awaken the Heart-Mind, there are specific methods and practices downstream that you can attempt. Without the active use of the Heart-Mind these aren't possible to accomplish.

You can obtain great benefits from intent. However, people with intent alone are not normally resolving their deepest psychological and emotional issues, and finding their sense of being connected to all of life. You're not going to find that genuine satisfaction arises solely out of intent. This is why some people clearly recognize their faults or "sins," but they are quite powerless to overcome them through conscious will or ordinary intent alone.

If human beings truly want to tap into something bigger than themselves they cannot do it without accessing the Heart-Mind.

You can make energy move through your body to gain certain benefits, but if you add the Heart-Mind into the mix, there's dramatically more that comes out of it. The Heart-Mind is what allows humans to integrate their experiences, and become smooth with them during practice and daily life.

Ordinary intent can make you a high performer at external tasks, but no more. What you will never achieve—no matter how much intent you use—is feeling whole inside. Ordinary intent will not make you smooth inside yourself. By its nature intent breeds the next intent because no intent can be complete. It always leaves you with what's missing. Integration occurs where everything comes together and where it truly is "all good." Something has to create continuity in your life, and accessing and opening up the Heart-Mind is a primary factor.

From an Eastern perspective, this does not only concern the mind. It's about the spiritual consciousness and deepest emotions that reside in the heart along with your rational capacity to figure out what's going on around you. For example, you can be completely at ease inside if your heart is open, but conversely you might not be able to walk down the street without getting lost if your intellectual mind functions poorly.

You don't need to have a Heart-Mind that's completely open to be more integrated inside. It's similar to the difference between being stark-raving mad, to being kind of okay, to being mostly okay, to being absolutely fine. Life exists along a continuum.

Bagua as the Heart and Soul of the *I Ching*

As a meditation art, a core principle of bagua is the Chinese concept of *bien hua* or "change." It is the heart and soul of the *I Ching*.

The Single Palm Change contains 10,000 energetic strategies of the *I Ching*, which provide insight into how one energy, event, situation or anything in existence changes into another. This is what happens when symbolically one or more lines in an *I Ching* hexagram changes from yin to yang or vice versa, and a new hexagram comes into being. The process by which one hexagram changes into another is called *bien hua*.

A core reason for practicing the Single Palm Change is to gain an experiential and visceral understanding of the processes of the *I Ching*. The practitioner seeks to go beyond mere intellectual understanding and explore the internal rules of change within universal energies. When you personally experience how chi changes inside your own body/mind, you also experientially gain insight into the self-evident ways in which chi governs external events and situations.

Through the Single Palm Change, you develop a personal interaction with the *I Ching*. By learning how to feel and directly perceive within your own body and awareness the various kinds of chi and energetic processes, you learn how to use the *I Ching* in your daily life to

- Initiate change
- Carry through and support change
- Facilitate change through its natural unfolding and prevent blockages if it freezes in place through inertia or unrecognized internal resistance
- Naturally or unnaturally terminate change.

Rather than just comprehend its intellectual meaning, the objective is to make the *I Ching* personally relevant and spontaneously applicable in daily life. It was for exactly this purpose that the Single Palm Change was designed by the ancient Taoists. Once you have a sense of bien hua, you gradually use the Single Palm Change in combination with the changing lines map provided by the *I Ching* for progressively more refined meditation purposes.

For example, within most external martial arts forms there is one formal, correct way in which a specific strike can be performed. If you wish to change the angle of your attack, you must use a different external form that employs a new desired angle. Bagua works differently. Using bien hua, you change the internal resistances inside your body, so it can appropriately adapt and instantly strike or defend at the new angle. This is done within its existing shape without assuming a new external form.

Likewise, you may find as you Walk the Circle that the energy of anger toward someone in your mind spontaneously arises. Using bien hua, you would change the manifesting energy of anger while still in mid-motion. You could neutralize the energy by perhaps changing speed or direction to hyperenergize your walking. Alternatively, you could change the energy of anger into the energy of compassion by supercharging your walking and, at the same time, projecting healing energy toward the person or situation for which you were angry. Anger—whether toward yourself or someone else—can create karmic suffering downstream.

Performing the physical movements of the Single Palm Change improves your ability to accommodate more powerful energetic flows and release the internal bindings of your soul or being.

BAGUA IS A LIVING ART

In the martial art style of bagua as taught by Tung Hai Chuan, there were about ten to fifteen basic form movements, which have been formally lumped together and called the Single Palm Change.

Tung, like a good tailor, adjusted the Single Palm Change for each student to best serve the specific needs of his uniquely individual body, mind and energy. Tung created a physical form suitable for many individual body types and chi structures to best experience bien hua, or the possibility of changing smoothly.

Sadly, through the generations, these variations on the palm changes have been codified into highly rigid forms. Some bagua schools go so far as to say that there is only one correct way to do the Single Palm Change. Of course, this is always consistent with the way their particular school practices it.

The better students of Tung passed down how these changes could be created or modified. Their students in turn created their own forms, which created their own innate bien hua movement forms. Liu Hung Chieh learned this art from one of Tung's main students.

This living tradition is what makes bagua a malleable, living art, comparable to a self-generating computer program that has many variations and permutations.

This is in distinct contrast to many external martial arts and qigong systems where the forms are often inflexible. The goal is to recreate the specific outer effect teachers have taught their students for many generations—even if they may not remember why the external forms were created in the first place.

The more you understand the inner meanings of the *I Ching*, the more you work with its principles to accomplish the goals of your meditation. This is true for clearing emotional demons as well as releasing psychic and karmic blockages. How you move and focus your attention, even in minute ways, changes the energies inside your body.

The subject of bien hua is also about how living beings, including humans, change and transmute over time. In bagua, these changes can occur over weeks, months or years with regard to formwork. However, ten changes in less than two seconds are also possible within more advanced meditation practices.

Bien hua is concerned with how your internal chi and body interact with and change each other. This is particularly true when you encounter a situation where your chi increases or instantly jumps to a higher level of capacity.

In bagua's spiritual or meditation aspect, bien hua is ultimately concerned with how you jump from one level of consciousness to another. You either resolve the blockages in your first six energy bodies or go beyond through internal alchemy practices.

Sadly, the study of bien hua is lacking in most Western bagua schools. In China's superior bagua schools, all principles are taught and practiced in terms of bien hua. *Hsing* or "form" is the specific pattern in which the body moves and the specific outer shape it takes. Hsing is the basis of external martial arts and qigong—not classic bagua.

Flexibility toward Change

I Ching meditation practices help you achieve the goal of being painlessly and appropriately able to change from one situation to the next. This fluid change may be within your own inner world or in relationship to other people or events. Meditation allows flexibility in how you react to situations of engagement and change.

Gaining awareness and adaptability to the natural flux of situations is gained through Circle Walking and, by extension, in your daily life. A primary directive of bagua and Taoist meditation is to seek naturalness in all actions, especially during changes. Using bagua and sitting meditation practices together works synergistically.

Even after learning how to physically let go at every moment of Walking the Circle, you may find that you still have some internal resistance that keeps you from progressing. Maybe you are still holding certain ideas of what you "should" be doing as you walk. Maybe you now need to let go of some concept on which you are still fixated. Releasing these fixations is not easy. However, continued bagua practice and sitting meditation can help fuse disconnected parts inside the brain and facilitate releases.

Bagua uses all sixty-four psychological and spiritual paradigms of the *I Ching's* hexagrams without being fixated on any one of them. Every time you use the Single Palm Change to reverse the circle's direction, you have an opportunity to explore one or more of those paradigms. In the flow, you can create change, wait patiently for change to come or allow change already in progress to complete itself in its own time.

Resolving Deeper Emotional Blockages

Much of what occurs in the early stage of bagua as Taoist meditation involves either actively or passively smoothing out the energies of deeper negative emotions. The tremendous twisting and spiraling internally and externally causes trapped emotions inside the body to spontaneously release. This is particularly true of emotions that are found deep within the subconscious and far below your levels of conscious awareness. Through bagua practice, emotions can be energized and come to the surface. From there they can be positively transformed by using specific methods of moving or sitting forms of meditation.

The emotional resolution methods of bagua and meditation are a part of what is commonly referred to in the *I Ching* as the process of changing the "inferior man" into a "superior man." From the Taoist perspective, almost all people are born inferior and only by applied effort or circumstances of great good fortune can they become superior people.

Initially, recognizing and taking full advantage of the exact moments during Circle Walking, when your deeper emotions become accessible, usually requires the input of a teacher's energy. Working with a book alone is not sufficient, as this is an experiential rather than an intellectual process. Input from a master can save years of wasted effort. Over time, a teacher's input enables you to recognize the critical moments when immense opportunity for change exists. Once the opportunity disappears, it might be replaced by an emotional wave. You have the best chance of successfully practicing on your own after studying this process with a master.

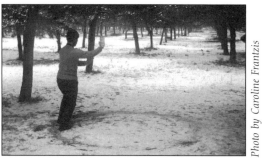

A bagua practitioner Circle Walking in a Beijing park wears a circular track in the snow.

Photo by Caroline Frantzis

When Walking the Circle, you may undergo altered states of consciousness. They may exist only for very short or intermittent periods before vanishing. A teacher who recognizes these moments as they happen can help bring about emotional resolution.

RELEASING ANGER

If you are Walking the Circle and realize—or you already know—that you have a habitual problem with anger, there are a few steps to dealing with it.

First, you have to recognize that the subtle emotion arising just below the edge of normal awareness is anger. You must investigate its energetic qualities. You then use Circle Walking and/or the Single Palm Change to more strongly activate the anger to enable you to access it inside you. Hovering on or just below the surface of your awareness won't be enough.

Perhaps you might be in doubt as to what you are feeling. Maybe it's there, but is it, really? You want to use your movements to get as much of that energy activated as humanly possible, not just five to ten percent, but much more so that you can no longer have any internal doubt.

Next, you sit quietly, go inside and apply the specific Taoist meditation methods you have studied. These could be Fire or Water methods of transforming or dissolving, respectively, to resolve that energy from a gross level to a more spiritual one.

After resolving the energy to the best of your ability, you Walk the Circle again—whether immediately or at the next practice session—to activate and gain more access to these deep energies within you. In this way, the flow between Circle Walking and sitting meditation becomes a continuous, unbroken circle.

Expanding the Mind

As discussed, an essential quality of bagua as meditation is expanding the nature of the mind so that you can focus on many things at once without getting polarized or fixated on one thing or expectation.

As your skill grows, the synergy of neigong techniques opens up your awareness. You might, for example, develop the ability to breathe extremely evenly and experience it moving very strongly through your internal organs. This action opens up the energy of your organs, which can help release the emotions frozen in your mind.

Since opening the mind helps release blockages and minimizes your tendency to be distracted, you're less likely to flip into the unconscious mind and trigger the subliminal memories that are stored there. Some of these memories can be incredibly stressful, such as the death of a loved one, divorce, childhood abuse, being in a war zone, or the sense of past failures or fear of success. When these memories are triggered, the mind contracts and becomes even more stressed and distracted—a nasty downward spiral. The antidote is to expand or open the mind using neigong.

Bagua teaches you practices to deeply feel how your mind contracts when it encounters stress. You must recognize the difference between consciously carrying out a task (for example, looking at your finger in the Single Palm Change) and the potential effects of the stress it may trigger in your unconscious mind. As your mind expands, you become much more present—eventually also tuning into the events happening below your normal conscious awareness.

In time and with practice, you can penetrate the barrier between the conscious and unconscious mind. This allows your conscious mind to expand into unconscious parts of your awareness that previously were closed to you. The repetition of going around and around the circle enables the breaching of this conscious-unconscious barrier through gradual dissipation. Walking the Circle is like walking around threshing and winnowing wheat to separate it from the chaff. Each time you go around, more of the wheat separates from the chaff. So too will you let go of what is stuck and frozen in your mind.

This is all part of the spiritual relaxation process of Taoist meditation. Although the barrier may remain intact for many years, you initially learn to accept its presence without agitation until it has less and less of a negative effect on you.

As your mind expands, you also progressively become aware of the energies and subtle phenomena both inside and outside you. You become less fixated on any particular energy or configuration of energies through the process. Your mind becomes receptive to all possibilities of change, which goes far beyond merely reducing stress.

Being at Ease in the World

Eventually, you will apply the knowledge you've gained about change from the *I Ching* and your practice of bagua into everyday life events. As you become more conscious of how events in your life change from one into another and liken it to the flows you constantly experience in your Single Palm Change practice, you learn to flow more smoothly with changes in your life.

Bagua meditation helps you develop the sense of being open to—yet not bound by—whatever events occur in your everyday life. Within that openness, that space, you develop the internal capacities to generate whatever state of mind you would like to have in your life. None of us can control outside events 100 percent of the time, but you can learn to manage how you respond to them. So, if you wish to be happy in the most adverse circumstances, you must generate happiness from inside yourself. You cannot rely upon external events, goals or expectations to make you happy. Winning the lottery or finding an ideal job probably won't solve your long-term emotional blockages. Likewise, being bound by negative events and not being able to move forward in your life will not foster health and happiness.

It is possible, through bagua as meditation, that your mind can become peaceful and find a complete ease with anything that's going on. As Lao Tse put it so eloquently, "Man of the Tao has no enemies."

Flowing and Finding Stillness

How can you flow with the changes every day brings and stay present within any maelstrom life chooses to send? This is the challenge of what you eventually progress toward as you practice bagua as an *I Ching* meditation method.

Equally important is: Can you flow with change without having an agenda? Sometimes changes happen that you are powerless to affect. And yet even in such situations, you still know the general direction of the flow somewhere inside yourself—even considering the unpredictable currents you may encounter.

A surfer who catches a tall, twenty- to thirty-foot wave in Hawaii might know the way that he'd like the wave to break, but he damn well can't make it happen. Like the surfer, you find the wave's flow as best as you can. You do the best possible. Your focus must stay on riding the wave, so that no matter how the wave changes, you can stay on it.

More ideal still is to reach a point in your practice where there ceases to be a distinction between you and the wave, or you and the circle you're walking. There's neither the wave nor you, only an event that is in play. If you can relax and let the event unfold into the unknown, this is where the magic appears.

The surfer is doing whatever is possible to stay on the wave. It also means the wave will do what the wave will do, and cares nothing about the surfer.

So the questions are: Can you open up enough and relax into the energies of the universe—where things manifest, come into existence and go out of existence? Can you find the center of all that change where you can just be? Can you find and anchor yourself in the unchanging empty center of the *I Ching* while allowing change to happen and simply being a part of it without resistance?

There is a place in the middle of the *I Ching's* eight trigrams that is unwavering and constant. In Taoism this is called the Tao, or emptiness. This place is utterly and totally free and leaves within it the potential for any kind of change to take place. The empty center permeates all change. It is melded to all change and yet itself is never affected by change. That is the fundamental principle behind the *I Ching* and the Taoist spiritual art of bagua.

Working with the Energies of Nature

Exploring your internal world can lead to understanding how your internal energies interact with the energies of the external environment. This begins with your immediate environment such as trees, grass and deep into the earth below you. It eventually spans huge distances—potentially including the planets and stars. This is yet another example of the sophisticated use of the *I Ching* map as applied to the practice of bagua.

At a practice level, you let go and move into a space that has nothing to do with you, becoming concerned only with an "event" occurring at that moment in time. Beyond what's happening within your own energy, there is equal concern for the energy of the surrounding environment. This includes the energy of the earth, stars, sky, trees and all the natural energetic forces surrounding you, and human manifestations like politics and economics. You allow your physical movements to harmonize with the matrix of environmental energies coming together. In time, you'll find pure joy in blending with the forces of nature.

Resonating with the energy of the earth is of particular interest from a Taoist point of view, since we are inhabitants of this planet. Like many traditions of the ancient world, Taoists believe the earth is a living being. Contacting and melding with the energy of the earth will help you naturally acquire the wisdom it holds.

As you become more connected to the energies of nature, your natural human capacities to connect to the intelligence of the universe follows. You realize that you are part of it and it is a part of you—a microcosm within a much larger macrocosm.

Pre-birth Practices

Meditation and the art of bagua share another particular focus, which is known as *Hsien Tien* or Pre-birth practices. These start with a simple question: Where do human beings come from?

Scientists might answer, "Their mother's womb, from a sperm and egg."

Taoists would say that it's a big jump from the fusion of a sperm and egg to a human being with its immeasurable consciousness. They pondered and asked other questions: When a human being is in its mother's womb, how does consciousness enter into the body? What allows it to grow the internal force that becomes its mind and immortal spirit?

Taoists believe the way a human being is energized while in the womb is different from the way he or she receives chi after entering the world. After birth, humans gain new energy through exercise, breath, food and rest. In the womb, cosmic forces charge up a baby like a storage battery. Much of the charge received before birth will be used later in life. Taoists say that the amount of energy initially stored in the "battery" of the womb will determine that human being's general constitution throughout its life span.

Taoist Pre-birth practices attempt to reconnect with the original cosmic forces to charge the human battery in the same way it was charged while in the womb. Effectively, they upgrade a person's basic genetics. Post-birth chi practices attempt to optimize what remains of a person's original pre-birth chi. You try to conserve that chi by maximizing the degree to which you can draw chi from other sources (exercise, breath, food and other factors in the environment).

The subject of how you can reconnect with the original force that came into you, developed and "charged you up" as a baby is the subject of the Pre-birth spiritual practices of bagua.

Pre-birth practices involve changing your body so that you can tap into the universal energy that you received externally while inside the womb. These techniques seek to resolve some of the more difficult karmic influences and needs that resulted in your birth and existence in a human form on this earth.

Pre-birth practices are intended to help you go through the layers of your consciousness and eventually arrive at the pure space from which you descended to the earth and into a body. This journey to the source may be unfamiliar unless you have some knowledge of the inner or esoteric traditions of the world's major religions (including Gnostic Christianity). This return journey is about the actual mechanisms of consciousness and is not normally taught within orthodox, belief-centered religions.

At its root, Bagua Circle Walking is a Pre-birth energy practice. The simple act of Walking the Circle creates a vortex, which allows the practitioner to amplify, mix and control the energies that naturally rise upward from the earth and descend from above (referred to as "heaven" in the Taoist tradition). Adding bagua's twisting actions further enables you to tap into your more refined energy bodies. Through the twisting movements you create spirals of these energies and the spiraling energies can involuntarily move your chi and body. Over time, you enable and direct vortices to simultaneously spiral within your body upward toward heaven and down toward the earth. This movement unravels the deeper mysteries of the human condition.

Tai Chi's Spiritual Exploration of Yin-Yang

In tai chi, the primary emphasis of practicing a form as an advanced method of Taoist meditation is to explore the nature of opposites, the nature of emptiness and non-duality. These are the concepts of tai chi and wu chi. This is practiced through tai chi's rhythmic alternation between yin and yang through slow-motion movement.

Tai chi as spiritual exploration also requires that you embark on three key stages toward achieving the goals of Taoist meditation:

1. Fully open up the energies of the body.
2. Purify any blockages in the emotional, mental, psychic, karmic or essence bodies using the methods of emptiness, to find out who you are beyond any personal history or identifications with the different aspects of your ego.
3. Learn to go beyond yourself and become simultaneously consciously aware of the universe (the Tao).

Rhythmic Movements

Tai chi as meditation is very strongly based on being exquisitely aware of the opening and closing motions within all the body's joints and cavities. The spaces inside your body at micro-levels rhythmically expand and condense in coordination with the retraction and extension of your arms and legs, known as "bend and stretch" in tai chi jargon.

While practicing tai chi's yin-yang rhythmic motions, a person seeks to find the center of stillness or emptiness. In this space, the yin and yang that are perceived as being opposites resolve into unified stillness, or tai chi.

Exploring Non-duality and the Underlying Nature of Opposites

Tai chi's main meditation goal is using movement to explore the Taoist principle of yin-yang. You seek the state or place where all seemingly opposite yin-yang qualities (e.g., night-day, high-low, good-evil and male-female) originate, exist, are the same and can cease to exist.

Any yin-yang pair at a deeper level implies several possibilities, such as
  • Yang (this)
  • Yin (or that)
  • Neither yang not yin (neither this nor that)
  • Both yin and yang (both this and that).

In tai chi, potential conflicts or disturbances that arise between any set of yin-yang opposites can be resolved, including a person's greatest personal traumas and highest aspirations.

The key is to find the place inside your mind where it does not get polarized into yin or yang—to tap into the Heart-Mind. In this space, you can fully accept both the yin and yang of anything: good and bad, this and that, up and down, forward and back, in and out. In this space your mind has no definitions and yet any definition can naturally come out of it—anything in any shape, manner or form.

The space of the Heart-Mind is classically described in Taoism and Buddhism with phrases such as, "Mind/no mind, form/no form." If you have a "mind," you can functionally use it to usefully comprehend differentiation. If you have "no mind," you're incapable of comprehending why any two thoughts could be in destructive or disharmonious conflict with each other in the first place.

Yet within the core of human awareness and mind/no mind, any two yin-yang thoughts can simultaneously and comfortably coexist. This is the tai chi space of your mind. You can experience it in the practice of tai chi as a meditation.

The specific spiritual terms used for many of these yin-yang resolutions are found in books on tai chi. In the English language, they can sound very strange, para-doxical and off-putting to the average Westerner. Some popular examples:
  • Form is emptiness, emptiness is form.
  • From stillness comes movement and from movement comes stillness.
  • To open is to close and to close is to open.
  • Seek the straight from the curved.

When tai chi is practiced as qigong, these yin-yang principles are explored in the context of your body and the relationships of the various types of chi within it. You track an incredible number of differentiations simultaneously and, over time, become aware of and seamlessly meld many yin-yang complements, including:

- The body's front and back.
- The right hand moving up while the left hand moves down.
- Arms are on top and legs are on the bottom.
- The spine opens one way and closes another.
- A given organ moves this way while another moves another way.
- Blood is directed to do this here and that there.

You can't reasonably expect to keep track of so many details without tapping into the Heart-Mind. In tai chi as meditation, you extend this approach into all realms of human experiences, from the emotional and mental to the psychic, karmic, and even to your essence.

Your goal is to find and recognize the tai chi place in your mind where these differentiations come together and become one simultaneously within emptiness.

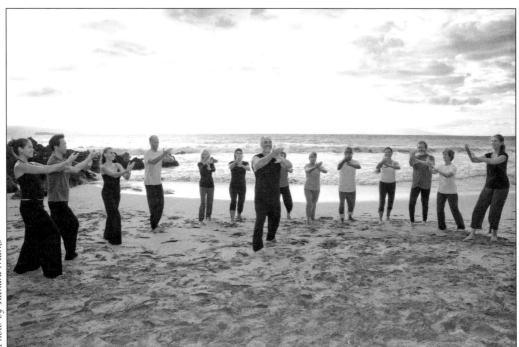

Photo by Richard Marks

The author and his students practice Wu style tai chi.

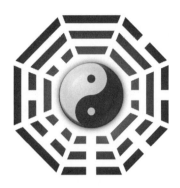

CHAPTER 10
Finding a Good Teacher

If your goal in practicing bagua or tai chi is to have fun, almost any teacher will do. However, if you wish to get the most out of these arts, training with a good teacher is paramount.

The three most critical criteria in finding a good teacher—in any subject—are that he or she:

- Is competent and has genuine knowledge about what is being taught.
- Knows how to teach.
- Is sufficiently clear and engaging so that you can understand and be inspired by the subject.

Finding a good teacher becomes even more essential for those interested in studying bagua and tai chi as something beyond physical exercise. Only a master can genuinely take you to the next level of learning how to use Taoist energy arts to develop chi and your spirit.

Not all teachers know the same material. Nobody can teach you what they personally don't know. Others may know the subject well, but can't teach it. A teacher who can do both is rare in any subject.

Just as certain athletic coaches consistently produce winning teams, so too do great teachers of bagua and tai chi consistently produce great students. Exceptional mentors inspire, spark and expand the artistic talents of the next generation of teachers and practitioners. Traditionally, masters and lineage holders in the energy arts are responsible for creating their counterparts in the next generation.

No matter how good the teacher, you must put in sufficient, sustained effort and practice time to achieve success from the seeds of your learning. In the chi arts, personal creativity, intelligence, talent, perseverance and intuition are needed to best learn and practice efficiently.

Teachers of Physical Arts

If your interest in learning bagua or tai chi is primarily as a physical art, several considerations are important when assessing a potential bagua or tai chi instructor. These are not unlike assessing coaches of most sports.

- Do they teach the basic foundations sufficiently? In addition, for the best results downstream, you want a teacher who helps you continuously improve even as techniques become more sophisticated or complicated.
- Do they teach safety protocols of how the movements should be done? These help protect you from damage downstream and hurting yourself unnecessarily. Although you won't know what these safety precautions are specifically, at least make sure that safety protocols are taught. With proper safety instruction, major problems almost never arise.
- Can you "vibe" with or at least respect the instructors sufficiently that you can accept their instructions without resisting them? Can they inspire you sufficiently to motivate you to practice on your own? This is a key factor in obtaining higher-level success in either bagua or tai chi. Good teachers will get you over humps when you get discouraged. If these qualities are not in place, you will most likely quit and thereby never get what you came looking for in the first place.

Teachers of Chi Arts

Most teachers of bagua and tai chi as only physical exercise will not commonly be of much help when you want to learn bagua and tai chi as higher arts of developing chi. Students will have to seek out teachers that know and can teach the arts of chi development or neigong. For most students, developing chi is a mandatory prerequisite to the genuine spiritual practices of Taoism.

Equally, if you want to learn the chi of the healing arts, then those teachers who have learned the chi of Traditional Chinese Medicine will be more effective at teaching healing than teachers of bagua and tai chi as physical exercise.

Teachers of chi are unlike teachers that teach from an intellectual or theoretical point of view. Most Westerners are used to teachers only intellectually explaining a subject and/or setting up rational experiments to clarify the premises being taught.

In the chi arts, teachers plant what you might call a seed of chi inside the students' bodies so they can absorb and begin to grow their own chi. Students have to be able to recognize and feel the qualities of chi inside themselves, which is not theoretical or intellectual.

Then, the absolutely necessary and specific techniques and methods the teacher imparts become like the fertilizer and water. Every seed requires sustenance to grow into a strong and healthy plant that can produce seeds of its own.

A teacher can't give you the chi they don't have. Only teachers who have strong chi within themselves can transmit it to you so you can get it in a concrete way. Some excellent teachers may also be logically organized; their teaching methods may be clear and systematic. However, in teaching and imparting the seeds of chi to settle within you, it is also essential that teachers impart it in a way that is beyond logic and thinking.

Teachers in some schools hold a few of the sixteen neigong seeds. Some hold many. Few know all the different types of energetic work that the original internal styles possessed. Having any of them will allow a teacher help you more, but the more they have the better.

Nevertheless, a teacher might have strong and brilliant chi, impress the hell out of you, but be unable to communicate or plant that seed within you in ways you can access, absorb and assimilate. Many students are not clear on this point and fool- ishly expect that any teacher should have that ability, which may not be the case.

Chi masters are in many ways like the masters of music. Some practice for God knows how long, can do everything technically right, yet when they play, the chi or sweet soul of the music just isn't there. Again, it's hard to give away what you don't have yourself.

With the best musicians, something about the way they play resonates and inspires their students, improving their performance by quantum leaps. These musicians have magic in the soul. The vibrancy with which they perform clearly arouses listeners deep inside.

In the chi arts, teachers have a range of styles and qualities which give their students access to understanding. The primary quality is their chi.

To complicate the matter, some masters have the abundant physical chi of small elephants, but not much in the way of the other two Taoist treasures: energy and spirit. They may also have severe human limitations in terms of their mind and emotions. For hundreds of years in China there was little shortage of ordinary bagua or tai chi martial art masters who were alcoholics, drug addicts or considered crazy in one way or another. Being a physically powerful and healthy alpha male ape does not necessarily mean that that person is emotionally and mentally coherent.

LIU TALKS ABOUT CHI

When I first met my teacher Liu, I announced that I wanted to get more chi. Liu laughed at me and said I had more than enough chi for a very large animal—definitely sufficient for any human needs.

Liu explained that spiritually it was my Heart-Mind—not my chi—that needed to grow. These are immensely important words for any bagua or tai chi practitioner.

The study of spirituality and the Heart-Mind are about intent and chi. The Heart-Mind is the key to what the Taoist internal practices, including qigong, bagua and tai chi, truly have to offer.

Teachers of Spirit

When systems of exercise are based on mind-body fusion, chi, spiritual work and meditation, the essential ingredient for success is to train with a genuinely qualified teacher. This is as true for bagua, tai chi and Taoist meditation, as it is for Buddhism, yoga and all authentic spiritual traditions of subtlety on this planet. Masters in these fields will use both use ordinary and esoteric methods of teaching.

In Taoism, developing the chi of the body is the first step in the process of converting chi to spirit. High-quality martial art masters of bagua and tai chi can usually teach the health maintenance and healing aspects of the energetic methods of Chinese medicine within the three treasures. However, generally this covers nothing beyond the body aspect.

If the issues you wish to resolve within yourself concern all the three treasures— body, energy and spirit—then you need a teacher who embodies those qualities. You must find a master in the spirit aspects of bagua and tai chi to completely learn the chi-spirit-emptiness-Tao practices.

SAFETY ISSUES

In the teaching of these arts, physical, emotional and psychological safety should be a primary concern. At the level of health, for example, the teacher must be concerned with making sure students don't injure themselves, not just in the moment but down the line. Beginning practices emphasize alignments, principles of turning and protecting the knees and, most importantly, the 70-percent rule of moderation.

Safety is equally primary when students are learning to develop chi and spirit and begin to clear some of the deeper blockages within themselves. Teachers must be aware of how different chi and spirit methodologies should and could be taught in terms of time, effort and level of capacity so the student has the optimum chance of achieving their desired outcome. They must be clear about what factors could inhibit or block success even if a student applies enough effort during practice.

Teachers must also be able to know how to correct damage on all levels when students have either been incorrectly taught or careless about heeding the safety warnings of their teachers.

Mind-to-Mind Transmission: The Heart of Taoist Teachings on Chi

The energetic and spiritual qualities of bagua, tai chi and the higher esoteric traditions have always passed nonverbally between teachers and their students to the next generation. The teacher—in what could be called telepathy—transmits what he knows from his own heart and being to the heart and being of the student. The purpose is to energetically and directly communicate the reality of what is being taught in a totally nonverbal fashion rather than only hinting at it in words or showing the outer surface of physical movement.

If the student is lucky, he or she will get it immediately; if not, the seeds are sown within the student and if the student practices, these seeds will manifest when his or her Heart-Mind has grown sufficiently.

Direct transmissions are the heart and soul of spiritual bagua, tai chi and Taoist meditation, as well as included within many aspects of Buddhist and Hindu meditation. These methods of direct transmission form a living link between the generations.

Without this critical component, all the intellectual information relating to the methodology of these spiritual traditions can never reach its full potential. This is because an intellectual description of what a food tastes like—no matter how well-crafted or inspiringly presented—is no substitute for the actual chewing and tasting of the real food. In a similar manner, the information of the Heart-Mind of a bagua or tai chi practice is incomplete without the student tasting, in the depth of his being, what the real thing is like. These transmissions form the internal landmarks so that students can then manifest those qualities by themselves through step-by-step work.

Tung Hai Chuan taught Ma Guei bagua's martial tradition this way, in much the same manner as my teacher Liu taught me. Moreover, when psychic energy is involved—the invisible energy that causes the body to function and forms part of the roots of human consciousness—Western logical methods of teaching are insufficient. The teaching of genuine spiritual topics commonly goes directly to experiences, which thought processes alone are incapable of intellectually comprehending.

Only at the level of the root of the mind can the complete meaning of many teachings be completely understood. Conversely, at the level of the intellect and the physical body, they can only be partially understood or ultimately distorted. That is why direct mind-to-mind transmissions are the most critical component of all the world's genuine living esoteric or mystical traditions.

The necessity of direct transmission is the reason serious students are so concerned with lineages; who taught whom, who studied with whom; who taught what to which student. Lineages reveal when a clear transmission was given and verified by the teacher as having been authentically accepted and manifested in the student. Traditionally, lineages would protect the integrity of the teachings, at least to some degree, by preventing those lacking genuine training from falsely making claims about their capacities.

Without a good teacher the transmission will be poor and this living force of mind and chi passed on from generation to generation will be absent.

The Nature of Liu's Mind-to-Mind Transmissions

My teacher Liu transmitted as I practiced Bagua Circle Walking. Liu also did similar types of transmissions for tai chi chuan, hsing-i chuan and qigong with me, each with their own unique internal content and flavor. These were everyday occurrences that happened regularly during my daily three-plus years of private training in Liu's home.

Liu's room was about fifteen feet long and eight to ten feet wide. Dominating one side of this rectangle was his desk and chair with a light switch above it, another chair and then a double bed. In the middle of the room was a round table, which Liu used for eating and above it, very near the foot of the bed, hung two long scrolls filled with calligraphy. Each was opposite the room's door. Another side of the room was occupied with a bookcase and a small pot-bellied coal-burning stove, the sole source of heat and fire for cooking. At night the only lighting was a single, naked low-wattage light bulb.

When we worked together the small round table was moved to the back of the room's rectangle, leaving approximately a six-foot-square open space in the middle of the room. All the forms of bagua either of us did were done with very tight steps in this extremely limited space.

When Liu first taught a movement, he would have me follow him. He would place my hands, feet and body in the correct position a few times. Then he would ask me to do it. As I practiced, Liu did one of three things:

1. He wrote in calligraphy with his back to me.
2. He sat with his eyes closed.
3. He sat facing me with his eyes open, watching me like a hawk and giving encouraging commands by gesturing with his hands, eyes or face.

If he was in the third mode, practice was relatively easy. I knew what he wanted and did my best to comply. The other two modes, however, were more akin to the mysteries of Taoism in terms of both chi and the mind.

The Result of Receiving Liu's Mind-to-Mind Transmissions

Energies would manifest inside my body like a living force, directing my body to move in specific ways. By directly following and expressing the chi that was spontaneously moving through my body as I performed the movements of bagua, I began to go through the different stages of chi development according to the principles of neigong. As I experienced and consciously comprehended one kind of chi flow, that energy transmission from Liu would then suddenly cease to spontaneously manifest inside me. I would then practice and practice until I could manifest those same energies within the movement with my own effort in a very clear, specific and precise manner.

Over months, this slowly transmuted from the indirect to the direct chi practices. This happened so that the three tantiens and channels gradually would open, giving me a pragmatic chi road map. The methodology spontaneously brought me to new, higher and deeper levels of consciousness and spirit.

Liu's transmissions, along with copious practice on my own, allowed me to internally stabilize the chi road map at profound levels of chi and spirit. At the end of every practice session, after following strict rules of the techniques of Circle Walking and palm changes, the session would conclude with a shorter period of spontaneous movement intermingled with the formalized changes of either the monastic or martial schools of bagua.

Through this living force of chi moving in my body, the 4,000 to 5,000 functional energy lines in the human body became dramatically more apparent than they had been in all my years practicing as a qigong tui na doctor of Chinese medicine. Additionally, chi flows changed and intermingled with each other as the qualities of inner light and emptiness dawned, along with higher stages of consciousness manifesting within the Heart-Mind.

Liu and Chinese Calligraphy

Whenever Liu practiced calligraphy, I knew it was going to be an exceptionally difficult practice session. One of the goals of calligraphy is for the artist to transmit chi through the brush strokes onto the paper. Taoist calligraphers were famous for creating magic talismans, which caused events to happen. Liu used his calligraphy like a talisman to manipulate the chi within the room and in me. The chi took on a surreal quality of density in my body and spirit.

The room's energy would change in a few minutes and this energy would come down in a way that felt like gravity had been increased ten times. My arms and body were being pushed down with a tremendous force, demanding that I mobilize energies to combat it or be crushed to the ground. It was as though energetic weights were attached to every bit of my body.

Likewise, the more I was able to withstand and relax sufficiently to counter the feeling of weight, the more this force would penetrate and make me consciously aware of what was happening to the physical tissues of my body, the chi within it, and inside my Heart-Mind including the spiritual forces that lived there. This penetrating energy would stretch the tissue of my body from the inside out.

Afterward I sometimes would notice that if Liu was repeating brush strokes, they were formed in the same way that my body was being externally and internally moved and manipulated—or you could say forced into assuming different shapes. Strokes upward, downward and sideways caused upward, downward and sideways physical movements, internal chi flows and movements of consciousness within my body and away from it. If I had not actually gone through this, I never would have thought it possible.

Moreover, these were not broad, cathartic, spontaneous, sloppy free flows of chi and body movement, but tightly controlled and highly precise movements. Liu would manifest these energies within my body, chi and spirit. He did this not only for physical effects, but also to help me purge negative emotions, such as anger and fear, from my being. This brought forth different aspects of higher consciousness.

The same thing happened again when Liu sat with his eyes closed. Occasionally, when I was simultaneously spinning around the room, doing complex foot and hand changes, not crashing into any furniture and my mind was stable enough, I could see Liu clearly. I would feel that he was again controlling my internal chi and physical movement with complete precision by tiny movements of his hand, torso or head.

Liu Imparts the Intellectual Framework

We would usually sit and practice Taoist meditation before and after each Circle Walking or tai chi exercise. After a sufficient period, sometimes days, weeks, months or years after I experientially understood how and for what functions the chi was moving, Liu would allow me to ask him about the intellectual framework of how the neigong system worked—both as separate pieces on their own and when integrated together. Some of the aspects Liu explained were how some pieces or techniques could or could not be interconnected and in which specific ways.

After Liu had been doing a specific series of Heart-Mind transmissions and I had coherently comprehended the chi processes following prolonged hard work, only then would Liu explain how these techniques and their results fitted into the Taoist tradition from multiple perspectives. These included health, healing, meditation, longevity, martial arts, the nature of spirit and the Tao, and how events manifest over time.

Liu's teachings on the *I Ching* provided the 5,000-plus-year historical context that led to the development of bagua. Emphasis was always toward the essence of a method in the context of the eight energy bodies and not so much the specific technique's A to B to C progressions, which Liu also used to illustrate larger energetic relationships.

Once the essence of a kind of chi was experientially understood in a concrete rather than vague way, Liu then taught me how to recognize and generate primary forms of chi. He also made clear the nature of how any individual primary energy creates useful applications, secondary variations and permutations. As a result, my perception became both more expanded and more subtle. I came to realize that the distinctions made in the West about how matter, energy, time and events change are somewhat arbitrary.

Planting the Seeds of Bien Hua

I personally consider myself immensely lucky to have met Liu and undergone this meditation-based Heart-Mind transmission training. The day before he died, Liu taught me the final Wu style tai chi transmissions and the final bagua hand posture. It was physically, energetically and spiritually the most strenuous practice I had ever undergone in my life. I believe that without the years of prior training by Liu that my body or mind could not have withstood it.

Being more tired than I had ever known possible, I told Liu that this practice took a lot out of me. Liu looked exhausted and replied that it took much more out of him. I only realized the immense compassion that Liu had demonstrated in providing the continuity of these arts for future students when I learned of his death the next day.

Liu opened my mind in these talks, provided energetic transmissions about bien hua (changes) and planted the seeds of change in me in that only years after his death began to make sense. Now, my life's work is sharing what I learned to bring about positive change.

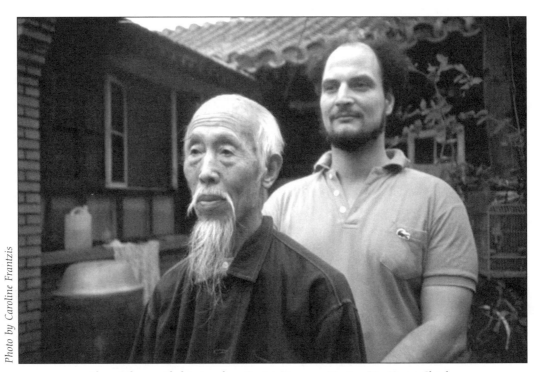

The author with his teacher, Taoist Lineage Master Liu Hung Chieh.

Conversations with Liu about Teaching in the West

Before returning to the West in 1987, I had many discussions with my teacher Liu in Beijing. I came to understand the teaching conditions I would most likely encounter upon returning home, especially in terms of students' learning capacities, time available to practice and accessibility to teachers.

It seemed that it would be virtually impossible to share more than the smallest percentage of the vast amount of material that Liu had so generously imparted during his one-on-one tutelage. We often joked that neither of us could be cloned.

Liu considered these constraints. After some months, he proposed a program that we discussed for many months. During these conversations, Liu brought to my attention perspectives that I probably never would have considered. He made the forest and the trees of his program's details completely accessible to me.

Liu advised, "First, consider that the original point of Taoism is based upon the idea of body-energy-spirit-emptiness-Tao"[1] (discussed in Chapter 3).

Phase 1: Body

Liu proposed that in the initial phase of my teaching, the primary consideration should revolve around all foundational methods relating to grounding and opening up the basic physical energies in my students.

The focus was to be on the body, including the necessary chi and meditation support. Above and beyond serving students' needs to learn the principles and practices that would enable well-functioning, whole-body integration, he felt the foundation should also include the chi work. This would help students become physically healthy and heal disease. He thought that if they wished to learn bagua

---

[1] He proposed that I roll out a program based on the three sections—body, chi and spirit (which includes emptiness and Tao)—each over a ten-year phase.

as a martial art, the foundational chi work could make them very strong. The body phase should include enough chi work so that students' emotional, mental and psychic life could become more smooth and balanced.

A minimum of meditation work would also be necessary for students to acquire a sufficiently solid foundation for the spirit to function well within the constraints of having a body. If in the future students wished to genuinely engage with the final phase of spirit through meditation, ideally, their bodies would need to be sufficiently prepared to undergo the rigors of Taoist meditation.

Phase 2: Chi

The next phase of chi goes beyond having students learn about the chi of the body (such as the energy channels of acupuncture), which is properly a part of the body phase. Rather the focus is on developing the chi of the emotions, mental thoughts and psychic realms. This is the foundation of sound emotional, mental and psychic health and creativity. If students lack a solid footing in the foundational work of the body phase, this work will go dramatically slower.

Many students might not quite understand what psychic health means because they will not have their internal senses or psychic body developed. Consequently, by the end of this phase, these qualities must be nurtured until they begin to function in a satisfactory way without undue strain.

The main task is to make sure students first become emotionally, mentally and psychically healthy. Next, they need to become very clear and finally very strong. Otherwise a perennial problem in the human condition could emerge. Until students' conscious, thinking minds and emotions can coordinate reasonably well, most will be rendered unable to understand the subtlety of the unseen world as it affects their emotions and rational mind. Most people will tend to deny the influence of the unseen world, particularly because of the fear of being personally unable to control it or being controlled by it.

Students must continually train to expand the supports of the body so that the energies of chi can move through their physical channels unimpeded. Otherwise, the body's energy channels can become clogged, which may have the potential to harm physical health.

Capacities of spirit (meditation) are also included so the mind can perceive with increased clarity what is happening to the student's inner world—without inaccurately distorting it. Work with spirit helps students avoid destabilization due to the qigong problem of "Fire Goes to the Devil." If chi practices are done incorrectly or in imbalanced ways the possibility exists that the body or mind can become ill.

Phase 3: Spirit

This final phase is called by many names, including spirit, mind, being, soul or that which continues after a person leaves the physical body behind. This quality lies at the very core of human consciousness and the third phase of practice enables human beings to experience it themselves.

Enhancing the health of spirit requires that students have the foundational support of body and chi. In this phase, Liu said that I should teach students what he had taught me in terms of entirely revamping the subtle qualities of the body's tissues and energy channels, in order not to inhibit the light and vibratory qualities of spirit from becoming healthy and awake.

In addition, Liu recommended that I teach students the methods that would upgrade the quality of their energy channels within their physical bodies. This would further support clarity and the health of their emotional, mental and psychic bodies. Meditation and spirit practices are taught with the greatest of care so that emotional, mental and psychic energies do not become unbalanced and warp the spirit.[2] The body, chi and spirit must smoothly and evenly become progressively healthier at each step along the way.

Specific challenges that Liu warned would require my special attention included how best to upgrade the energies of the body so that they would not prevent students from becoming conscious of their spirit. The body could be a potential obstacle, deadening students to their spirit. He added that care must be taken as the spirit becomes ever more bright. Otherwise, whatever a student has previously done to their body might prevent them from realizing that they are more than their body alone. The aim is to have a smooth flow between spirit, chi and the body where each one enhances the others.

---

[2] If you have any psychological or medical problems, you should consult your doctor or other healthcare professional before starting any new exercise or meditation program. Meditative practices, such as Taoist meditation, may not be suitable for everyone, and are not recommended for those with severe psychological conditions.

Teaching Spirit and Meditation

In conversations with Liu, I shared with him my lack of confidence in being able to competently share his teachings about spirit. To me, teaching neigong for the health of the body was not the same thing as applying it for healthy emotions, thoughts and psyche. This was my experience in working with students during the previous twenty-plus years where I had primarily taught martial arts and healing. I recognized that teaching body and energy was significantly different from teaching the spirit aspects, which entailed much greater responsibility and competence.

Liu considered what I said for quite some time. Then he said, "Let's meditate together," which we did for a long time. Afterward Liu said, "I understand your honest concerns." He explained that it might be quite possible that he knew me better at that point than I knew myself. It was his opinion that in time I would handle the task quite well. He said it was fine if it took me a little while to grow into a way of doing things. He advised me to take my time and mull it over, and when the time arrived and I was relaxed and willing, to go forward with his blessing and do so with confidence.

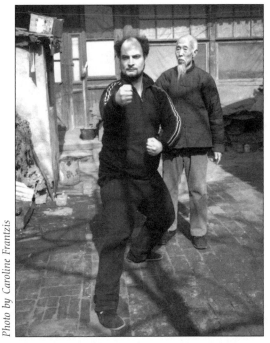

The author demonstrates bagua's Thunder Palm Change with his teacher Liu.

Later, Liu began to constantly tell me that my greatest talent would be teaching meditation and he thought it would be a really good idea if I did so after returning home.

At that time, I was in my mid-thirties and had already taught thousands of students since the age of fifteen. It's common for many who practice intensely and professionally for more than twenty years to think, "Well, maybe it is time to change, do something different."

When I mentioned this to him, he replied, "Why don't you teach people meditation? From what you learned before you met me and from what I can see you have learned now, you have enough to share with people that would be good for them. As a Taoist lineage master, I say you can do it without thinking you are unqualified."

Then he added, "Although you don't really understand now, because you have focused primarily on teaching martial arts and healing, you don't yet quite realize that your greatest talent will ultimately be to work with people's spirit. You don't recognize that talent, but I do and I think it's very clear."

Then in a very gentle, grandfatherly way, Liu continued, "On a practical level, you have explained to me how expensive proper teaching spaces for bagua and tai chi are in America, so meditation can be a solution. Consider you can get a lot more people in a room if they only sit in a chair rather than move around."

After considering Liu's advice, I told him I would think about it. I wasn't really up for it. My experiences with spiritual communities in the West and India had made me very familiar with the dysfunction I would have to deal with. Liu offered his understanding, but suggested that my compassion might grow. In that case, he thought I might find it less of a problem.

Then I explained that there were much better qualified teachers than myself. At least with martial arts and healing, I felt I knew what I was doing. Liu ended that conversation with a long "Hmmm … "

A few days later, Liu sat me down and said, "Although it may be true that you are not a Taoist Immortal, still, you know a little bit about how the Heart-Mind works. That's more than many. In addition, you are a good, experienced teacher. Don't worry—you'll do fine. I can understand how you feel this way. So until the time that you are willing to teach meditation, you don't have to. Just remember when you do feel it is okay, do it with my blessing. Please go ahead."

After some time had passed, I had a breakthrough, which I wrote about in my first meditation book[3] where I genuinely began to get a clear sense of the seventh energy body (the body of the Individuality), which Liu verified.

---

[3] See the author's book *Relaxing into Your Being*, Chapter 8.

Sometime after this Liu said, "Again, I would encourage you to teach meditation. At least you know who you are at the level of essence, which is more than many. So maybe it's a good thing if you teach … yes?"

I agreed, but with hesitation. Then, as I thought of the memorable meditation masters I had known, I added, "I don't feel like I really know what I'm doing."

Liu then said, "In this one sense, until you become a Taoist Immortal, you probably will never feel you know what you're doing. The fact that you don't feel that you know what you are doing doesn't show that you are humble. It shows that you are sensible and at least not completely self-deluded."

Liu repeated, "If you are willing, go ahead. If not, it's okay. You don't have to."

At which point I said, "Okay."

Teaching in the West

Liu's advice was extremely prescient. He anticipated and laid out almost everything I've personally encountered in teaching when I returned from China. He got to the heart of all sorts of issues that I could never have imagined.

What was especially perceptive was his advice to pay careful attention to the nature of what actually happens when people start opening up from the inside in real time. He gave me effective tools to prepare students so they could have a smoother, rather than a bumpier ride.

During the mid- to late 1990s, something inside me shifted. My sense of compassion for or maybe understanding of people in the West reached a tipping point. I realized that I although might not be the best in the world at teaching meditation, there was a lot I could do to help people.

So the tide turned and with it my willingness to teach meditation grew, which has only increased since the turn of the millennium. Meditation was always my deepest personal interest, and I'm of the opinion that it is probably the most important reason I went to China in the first place. It is the most valuable treasure that I brought back with me.

My early teachings centered primarily on the first phase of body practices: upgrading students' health and helping them acquire chi. I also included some of the second phase (energy) and foundational meditation work in preparation for the third phase (spirit) downstream.

My interest now is in helping to free human beings from that which is within their mind and spirit—everything that binds them—from the inside out.

APPENDIX A

Bagua for Lifelong Health and Maximum Performance

The development of chi flow can be considered in the context of bagua practice at varying stages of life.[1] Three interlinked aspects are considered:
- How the body ages
- What can be done to mitigate any negative impacts on the body and mind at each stage of life
- How best to help fulfill the natural needs of each stage of life.

The age ranges mentioned in each stage of life are approximate, not absolute, given the incredible rage of human genetic variation. What might apply for one teenager, might apply to another at twenty-two or twenty-three. Or, as baby boomers like to say: Yesterday's fifty is today's sixty or seventy.

Ideally, the following discussion of the aging process is about how to improve the quality of life, chi and health, allowing for a lot of variation as to how any individual might actually feel and experience the aging process. This is naturally highly subjective. More objectively, the practice of bagua will help you become less prone to ending up with medically-defined diseases as you age, or at least lessen their severity.

Stress Management

Learning bagua when you are young helps develop the strength and chi reserves to manage stress as you age. This is important because stress on the nervous system increases as you age and becomes increasingly precarious to your health.

This is why the American Medical Association states that the major cause of modern disease is prolonged stress. As the speed of mental activity increases, the nervous system can deteriorate, deplete the body's chi and tear the body apart.

---

[1] The author's book *Tai Chi: Health for Life* looks at these same issues from the perspective of tai chi.

Chi helps you withstand stress and thrive during it. Stress in your youth will deplete your chi later in life if you don't build up sufficient reserves to spend later. These energetic reserves commonly have three sources: abundant genetic strength, which either you are or are not born with; energy exercises like bagua or another powerful physical fitness program; and access to good food, clean air and water.

Generally, by the late twenties, the stressful adult world can hit you with the force of a hurricane. The need to have a life tool like bagua to handle tension reasonably well becomes a necessity for maintaining quality of life and good health.

By your thirties and forties, your professional life is often nothing but a constant assault on the nervous system. By then, if you haven't already learned how to deal with tension reasonably well, you'll really need a powerful form of stress-busting exercise, such as bagua. The effects of not being able to effectively deal with stress can fall on you like a house. You burn out more quickly, get sick more easily and take longer to recover than you did when you were younger. This is the time that many people begin developing chronic diseases, such as arthritis and diabetes. These are wake-up calls showing how stress can damage your health.

In your fifties and beyond, heavy stress may already have caused physical and emotional health problems, so you need to find a way to prevent them from dramatically worsening as you age. Many older people make statements like: "If I knew I was going to live to be sixty-five, seventy-five or eighty-five, I'd have taken better care of myself."

From your forties onward, managing stress merges with the desire to have peace of mind. Although this need for peace is more acutely felt at different ages, most mentally healthy people without drug habits, who have worked for two decades in high-stress environments, usually consider peace of mind to be increasingly valuable as time goes on. Peace of mind is one of the main reasons people practice meditation within bagua, tai chi, Taoism or other religious traditions.

When to Begin Learning Bagua

The ideal is for kids to begin bagua in their early teens and develop a lifelong practice to enhance adulthood and old age. Few younger kids will have the discipline and drive to practice on their own. In the modern era, pushing a child to do real internal work rarely succeeds. Kids must come to bagua of their own free will rather than through the relentless pushing of an older relative, no matter how well-meaning. It's best to simply encourage kids to go to classes and let them evaluate for themselves whether they want to continue.

Before children hit their teens, it is important that they strongly develop their muscles through such common physical activities as running around, climbing trees, biking, sports and martial arts like kung fu or karate. Vigorous exercise is essential to acquaint children with their muscles and enable them to naturally express the emotions that derive from normal physicality. It helps them fully develop energetically as they grow up.

Whatever stage of life you begin bagua, it can make you incredibly healthy and serve as a means for cultivating abundant chi. The point is, you get more benefits if you start bagua earlier rather than later in life. However, what is equally true (and somewhat miraculous) is that no matter when you begin learning bagua, it has the capacity to improve and keep improving your health and to reduce and keep reducing your stress.

Teenagers: Building Chi and Strengthening the Nervous System

Bagua helps teenagers grow strong bodies and powerful chi reserves.

Today, many teenagers don't get enough exercise and few are really fit. By the age of twelve, many kids already spend most of their free time watching television and playing computer games. They don't go out to the woods, climb trees, hike, bike or participate in sports. Many are not able to run a mile.

It is unfortunate that statistics show obesity among children and teens is increasing, and along with it diseases, such as diabetes and cardiovascular disease. The reasons most often cited are lack of exercise and poor diet.

If teenagers are to grow strong, they need a regular physical activity program that strengthens their bodies and their chi.

Particularly essential is that somewhere between the age of twelve to twenty-five, young people must train and strengthen their muscles and, to a lesser extent, fully develop their ligaments to avoid injury later on as they approach middle age.

Bagua is an ideal exercise for this purpose. It effectively works the muscles in coordination with the chi techniques that nourish, balance and strengthen them. It is challenging and aerobic in nature. Youngsters commonly enjoy its martial arts aspects. Most importantly, it gives them the opportunity to build a strong body and achieve lifelong health.

Without a strong exercise and chi-strengthening program, such as bagua, people can burn up their body's core energetic reserves at a young age. If they are already in energetic debt early in life, diminished from the get-go, this may leave them unable to withstand long-term stress in later stages of life.

Steadying Your Nervous System and Spine

Bagua teaches teenagers long-term stress management skills at the best stage of life to yield lifelong survival skills when they reach the modern work jungle. They have the free time and the natural enthusiasm of youth to develop those skills with maximum ease before the demands of life radically squeeze their time and energy.

Bagua develops a smoothly functioning nervous system that helps to manage the anxieties of teenage years. School demands can make many kids very hyper and anxious as they attempt to please their peers, parents and teachers.

Smoothly functioning nerves require a well-functioning spine. If spinal vertebrae are misaligned, it not only causes pain, but also scrambles the nerve signals to and from the spine. Both problems create nervous system stress and exacerbate stress derived from external events or inner psychological pressures. Weak or traumatized muscles and ligaments attached to the spine cause vertebrae to misalign. This is as much of an issue for youth as for older people.

Poor genetics, birth and other childhood traumas, or bad posture while spending long hours in front of a computer, can set the stage for back problems later in life. A spine made strong during the teenage years can make all the difference. A healthy spine will make it easier to recover from accidents in middle and old age, such as car accidents, falls and sports injuries.

From high school though graduate school, many teens and young adults often don't get more than four or five hours sleep a night, which can play havoc with the nervous system. The early start of high school classes may not accommodate teenagers whose brain physiology (biological clock) is telling them to go to bed very late and wake up late in the morning. According to the National Sleep Foundation, almost 80 percent of adolescents don't get the recommended amount of sleep. [2]

Bagua's ability to help keep the output of the nerves sufficiently steady and stable without becoming jumpy is especially helpful for high achievers during high school and college.

Bagua can help teens avoid the excessive, seemingly crazy behaviors and emotional roller-coaster rides that often lead to energetic depletion in their thirties and beyond. Practice helps youngsters burn off the stress and raging hormones that naturally create an immense amount of physical energy coursing through their systems. Bagua can productively channel this energy into a positive rather than a negative direction and smooth out spikes in hormone levels.

Bagua can help teens get rid of powerful negative emotions before they become deeply embedded and less accessible. The earlier they start learning how to achieve emotional balance, the more effectively they will be able to deal with setbacks later in life, for example, avoiding destructive or addictive behavior.

Twenties: Developing a Healthy Body

According to qigong medical theory, there are optimal times to develop different bodily systems so that they function with maximum efficiency throughout life. Knowing this will help you understand what deficiencies you may need to compensate for when you start bagua and other energetic practices later rather than earlier in life.

Strengthening Ligaments, Tendons and Fasciae

Before the age of twenty, physical strength primarily derives from muscles. After this, a shift occurs where significantly more strength derives from your ligaments and tendons.

Ligaments and, to a much lesser extent, tendons store subliminal emotions of which most people are not consciously aware. Deliberately developing and strengthening your ligaments and tendons enables stored subliminal emotions to be energetically cleared. Bagua accomplishes this rather brilliantly. If you energetically clear out

---

[2] National Sleep Foundation. "Teens and Sleep." www.sleepfoundation.org/article/sleep-topics/teens-and-sleep.

these emotions and stabilize your ligaments and tendons, this helps you avoid the unhealthy effects of getting older and the increasingly negative effects of stuck emotions as you age.

It is equally essential to get your fasciae in good condition. This is the connective tissue that binds muscles, tendons, ligaments and internal organs together. Keeping your body's fasciae flexible—smooth, moving and not flaccid or stuck together— makes a difference as you age. Damaged fasciae can start literally shrinking your body down, which can cause all sorts of physical problems, such as bad backs and tight shoulders. Moreover, if enough weakening or displacement of the fasciae occurs inside the abdominal cavity, problems may arise from internal organs becoming displaced and improperly aligned.

Bagua helps lengthen the body's soft tissues while your limbs extend and retract, deliberately stretching, unbinding and opening up the body's fasciae—not only around the big muscle areas (back, arms, legs, etc.), but also inside the abdominal cavity. Within the abdomen this allows ligaments and blood vessels to move and not be pushed upon or impinged. When the fasciae tighten around a place in your body, it impedes free movement or freezes the ability of other anatomical body structures to move within their natural ranges.

It is particularly important to strengthen the diaphragm, the massive band of fasciae just under your ribcage that rises and falls as you breathe, causing air to enter and leave your lungs. The diaphragm mechanically keeps you breathing. In the same way your diaphragm moves, so goes your breathing for good or ill. The diaphragm is also linked through an infinite number of anatomical interconnec-tions to your ligaments—strengthening these will help ensure that your diaphragm moves smoothly as you breathe.

Strong ligaments, tendons and healthy fasciae give you a physical superstructure that over your life span enables your body to move around doing your daily activities without restriction. You will be less prone to
- Joint or back problems—a bane of later life for most Westerners
- Easily getting injured
- Your breath weakening over time.

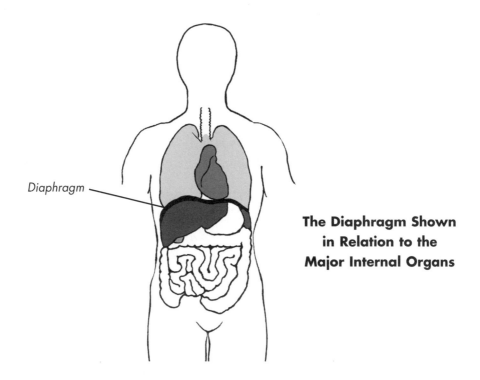

Diaphragm

**The Diaphragm Shown
in Relation to the
Major Internal Organs**

Regulating Hormones and Glands

If you learned bagua as a teen, you would likely have noticed that it helped prevent your hormonal swings from wreaking havoc. Without doing this kind of practice, by the time you are twenty and without parental constraints, the swings might tend to get more excessive. You now have the freedom to dance unrestrictedly all night long, drink coffee and alcohol in vast amounts and party for seventy-two-hour stretches.

However, with this freedom comes the tendency to burn out the body. Although the adrenaline rushes will make you feel as though you have a lot of energy for excessive behavior, it will cost you later in life and leave you at risk for body damage. These rushes pull and burn up chi from all your body systems and weaken your internal organs.

Bagua helps you regulate your glands. When you learn how to work with your glands and keep them functioning well, at each later stage of your life, you are best able to self-regulate them as appropriate. When you reach the more heavy stress periods of your life, not only can your glands produce what is necessary, but they can function in a smooth manner. This helps avoid hormonal peaks and troughs that would exacerbate the damage of any high-stress period in your life.

If you don't train your body to overcome or mitigate hormonal explosions, you may experience even more radical, excessive consequences. These may include erratic sleep patterns, binge drinking, drug addiction, outbursts of uncontrolled anger or depression. These problems may be avoided if you learn to smooth out the functions of your hormones with bagua as well as other chi practices.

Learning to regulate your hormones and glands will also help you create a significantly strong degree of internal cohesion. This in turn can enable you to recognize, rather than ignore or deny, how much stress your body is able to take before damage begins. You simply won't take part in activities that destroy and shred your body systems.

Strong internal focus is easier to create within yourself while the strength of the body supports it—in this case in your twenties, when the body's hormones are still running quite high. Bagua's Circle Walking begins to remove the barrier between the conscious and unconscious mind. As this barrier lessens, you become increasingly and consciously aware that *something* subliminal, *something* from your unconscious mind is driving you toward excessive behaviors.

Simply becoming aware and experientially recognizing what's going on—even slightly or at the unconscious level—can put a brake on any destructive behavior. By practicing bagua as a counterbalancing force, you can recognize when you are going over the top. The knowledge alone holds a lot of potential power and helps you naturally slow down negative tendencies rather than escalate them.

Thirties: Establish Strong Breathing Patterns and Optimal Circulation

The procrastinator's mantra is: Always put off until tomorrow (or never) what is most valuably done today.

By your thirties what you do (or don't do) really matters. The natural and abundant health gifts of youth will be gone unless you do something about them. You can make mistakes before the end of your twenties, blow them off and say to yourself,

"Oh well, I've got the rest of my life to clean them up." However, by the time you hit your thirties, you're moving into, "This is going to be the reality of my life." Most of the leeway or slack in your system will be used up and gone.

When most people approach or pass their prime, usually in their late twenties to early thirties, the natural energetic tendency is for their cardiopulmonary system—breath, oxygen absorption capacity and the ability to pump blood well—to diminish. Where there is blood you will find oxygen, nutrients, and life.

The counter to this effect of growing older is to establish strong breathing patterns to help weather life's increasingly stressful storms.

If you haven't done anything previously, your thirties is a critical point to develop your breath. After this the natural cycles of work, family and social obligations increasingly burden your system and can start corroding heart and pulmonary functions, just like strong acid corrodes metal. Establishing good breathing patterns is essential to increasing and maintaining a high level of energy, vitality and better blood circulation into your old age.

As you move into the later years of your life, it becomes extremely obvious that your ability to reduce stress and its damage becomes important. From your mid-twenties or beginning of your thirties to your forties, getting your blood and breath together is critical as both are dramatically affected by stress by the time you arrive at midlife.

As stress increases, many people stop breathing well and often involuntarily hold their breath. During longer work stints, their system may lack enough oxygen due to poor breathing. This can impair blood circulation and may increase the likelihood of heart attacks once people pass their thirties.

Bagua is one of the strongest ways to build a strong vascular system, upgrade your breathing and ward off heart and circulation problems.

Forties: Upgrade Your Internal Organs

If you reach your forties healthy, but still do not have a strong personal exercise practice, it becomes very important to "get it on" with a program that over the next twenty years will provide you with three major benefits:

- Strengthen your internal organs and significantly increase the chi flow between them
- Strengthen your spine to help avoid back problems later in life[3]
- Make your body as balanced and strong as possible

Bagua can give you these three gifts of life that will lead you to live more happily and healthily as you move toward old age.

The Chinese believe that an important benefit of bagua is to help your internal organs become healthier. According to the tenets of Traditional Chinese Medicine (TCM), internal organ malfunctions are ultimately responsible for most physical diseases. Organ malfunctions usually start arising after about the age of thirty-five, but it is usually only after fifty that the major diseases begin to proliferate.

Type 2 diabetes is common from about the age of thirty-five, whereas heart attacks become more common in those over fifty. Likewise, digestive problems start appearing more frequently around the age of forty.

Bagua's constant twisting and turning motions help create space within the abdominal cavities. This prevents all the anatomy inside from becoming constricted or restricted, allowing the internal organs to move freely and well. Bagua also facilitates all the natural physical and energetic interchanges between your internal organs, valves, blood vessels, ligaments, membranes, fasciae, and everything holding your internal organs together.

Bagua's constant turning actions twist and release the bindings between your internal organs. This in turn strengthens and tones them, just as normal activity and massage does for muscles.

This internal twisting inside the abdominal cavity also promotes better blood circulation between the internal organs and creates pressures inside the intestines, which helps regularize urination and bowel movements. By the time people reach their forties and fifties, urinary and bowel problems are common. Once they hit their sixties, having a regular bowel movement can become as important as sex was in their twenties.

---

[3] Bagua's twisting motions are not recommended for people who already have back and joint problems. Tai chi is better for those with injuries, but always check with your doctor first to make sure tai chi is suitable for your specific condition.

Why is this energetic emphasis on working on your internal organs from the forties onward so important? You don't end up in a hospital because your biceps or chest muscles aren't big enough or, if you are a woman, because your breasts are too big or small or your legs are not pretty enough. Hospital time usually arrives because your liver, heart, kidneys or digestive system malfunctions.

A weak spine is often a precursor to potential internal organ dysfunction. Internal organs hang off the spine like clothes on a hanger. If they hang poorly, problems often arise. This hanging of internal organs is visible in the swinging bellies of cows whose spines are horizontal rather than vertical like humans. So when aging human spinal vertebrae are unstable or improperly aligned consistently over time, this creates pressure on your internal organs.

Just as improperly hung clothes cause creases, internal organs hung poorly from the spine (and everything attached to it) absorb potentially harmful pressure. This can result in internal creases that cause health issues. The neigong spinal techniques within bagua are ideally suited to relieving this pressure.

Fifties: Preparing for Old Age

Your fifties can be the most active and productive phase your life. You have the accumulated experience to get things done well and still have the energy to pull it off. In terms of your body and chi, this is the time of life when you must prepare for old age or later suffer the unpleasant consequences of not having done so.

Nevertheless, in today's world of medical advances, what you do in your fifties or sixties and where you end up ten years later, will often be affected by whether or not you have financial access to the cutting edge of medical technology. Some procedures can get quite pricey. You could think of bagua as an extremely inexpensive health insurance policy.

Between the ages of forty and sixty the production of hormones begins to diminish. Yet to a certain degree, a person's general health depends on the natural energetic functioning of their glands. Both bagua's twisting actions and especially how it works with the central channel strengthen the glands of the body. This enhances most bodily functions and directly affects how the body and mind work and feel.

Large numbers of Chinese practice bagua and tai chi as a way to regenerate their sexual health. These arts increase libido, and the capacity to feel sexual pleasure and engage in lovemaking activity. In the West, sexual decline is thought to be linked to hormonal changes. In Chinese medicine, the weakening of sexual health is considered to be a consequence of a parallel weakening of the body's general overall chi, especially regarding the kidneys and nerves. Bagua and tai chi can be most effective for resolving these issues.

Stress and frustration can create adrenaline surges. If glandular secretions of adrenaline become strong and frequent, serious problems may result. Adrenaline surges combined with pent-up negative emotions, such as anger and resentment, can cause you to explode in ways that shake you up. These outbursts set the stage for high blood pressure and heart attacks.

For these reasons you must take strong actions to mitigate adrenaline surges by continuously maintaining focus on relaxing the inside of your body and calming your mind. This alone makes it worth the effort to learn bagua's Circle Walking and meditation methods. These practices can provide an antidote for an agitated mind that is unable to be at rest, function smoothly or sleep well. Otherwise you may become so contracted that you easily fixate on disturbing and potentially destructive emotions. Excessive frustration and anxiety can tear you down, burn you out and put you in the hospital.

If you haven't learned how to keep your mind calm and emotions smooth by the time you reach your forties or fifties, it's important to take stock of yourself and begin taking steps to make positive change.

Bagua includes a major emphasis on methods to Walk the Circle to activate and boost hormones and regulate the output of your glands, as do in different ways all Taoist forms of breathing, yoga and qigong. More advanced methods deliberately and strongly rely on

- The sixteen neigong components, especially working with the central channel
- Teaching you to consciously use your mind and physical movement to change the internal pressures inside the body in specific patterns.

A pragmatic emphasis on the central channel and chakras to help regularize the output of your glandular system is also part of the more advanced levels of classic Hatha yoga.

If you want to live joyfully as an older person, it is extremely important to make the glands strong to help bring you back to the kind of glandular strength you had in your twenties or thirties.

Sixties and Beyond: Regenerate the Body

In older age, the biggest issue is to avoid grinding down to a halt, physically or mentally. Someone who could go hiking for hours might end up barely being able to climb the stairs. A person's mind might become exceedingly rigid, incapable of letting go of even the most minor issues. You want to retain your flexibility and the ability to creatively and smoothly shift between ideas without becoming severely fixated or losing your way.

Bagua's Circle Walking can increase the circulation of fluids and plasticity within the brain. The constant, relatively rapid reversing of the circle's direction with various coordinated hand movements generally has a stronger and more powerful affect on stimulating the brain than tai chi.

From the sixties onward, bagua's greatest value is its ability to regenerate the body. You can attain the functionality of many forty-year olds. Although I have never personally seen someone revert to a twenty-year-old body, I have repeatedly seen those who are in the sixty- to seventy-five-year-old range bring back their bodies functionally to the point that of someone in their late thirties to early forties.

This always occurred through the mechanism of strengthening the chi of their system to a dramatic degree (often in combination with hsing-i or tai chi). This regeneration process can be very successful if the 70-percent rule of moderation is adhered to and you use very gradual approaches to training. At advanced stages of life, the more thorough and methodical you are in your approach, the faster the body can regenerate. Lifelong bagua practitioners, who may have used the 80-percent rule their entire life, should dial back and only do 70 percent, even though they may be capable of 80 percent.

Bagua for All Stages of Life

The beauty of the Taoist energy arts, such as bagua, is that they can engage and inspire you for life, whatever their intended purpose.

The power of chi is deeply transformative. Nourishing your chi will make you healthier and more relaxed for the rest of your life, well into old age. Bagua clears the physical blockages and negative emotions and thoughts, bringing back the joy and spontaneity you had as a child.

Bagua will help you connect strongly to yourself. If practiced as meditation, it will enable genuine love and compassion for yourself and others to flow naturally. As you open up to your human potential, the deep positive rhythms of the universe will come to your aid.

Chi practices can inspire you for the rest of your life. One of the most magical qualities I have found is that they continue to interest, engage and teach me new lessons, even after more than four decades of daily practice. They can do the same for you.

APPENDIX B

Why Buddhism and Hinduism Are Well Known, but Taoism Is Not

All branches of Buddhism and Hinduism came out of India, regardless of whether they ended up in Tibet, Southeast Asia or even Africa. Both religions carried the Indian perspectives on reincarnation and the idea that relationships between the individual and the collective soul or consciousness are linked completely and inextricably.

Taoism is uniquely Chinese.

India: Easy to Access for 2,500 Years

Westerners know so much more about the Indian perspectives of Buddhism and Hinduism in all their variations because they had the ability to go to India since the time of Alexander the Great, either over land, following the military routes of Alexander, or by boat from Alexandria to Southern India. Trade between the West and India was established from those early times and was accelerated when the British occupied India many hundreds of years ago.

From that time, some Europeans completely immersed themselves in what was for them a "new" spiritual culture. They learned written and spoken forms of the Indian languages, including Sanskrit and especially Hindi, and sought out spiritual and cultural leaders to teach them about these religions in their purest, clearest and most authentic—rather than distorted—forms.

When these travelers returned to their European homes, they could spread this knowledge in ways that made sense inside their own culture. They also brought over spiritual leaders who helped these religions flourish in fertile new soil.

This cross-fertilization occurred for many hundreds of years and continues strongly today.

China: Difficult to Reach, Hard Language and No British Empire

China was a different story. Before the 1800s few people traveled regularly to China and those that did were mainly Muslim traders, either traveling by boat or via the Silk Road between the Middle East and China. They went only for trade and profit and brought little back that would not bring them money. Translating texts of Taoist religious doctrines was not considered a high priority in Muslim countries. This is why the travels of Marco Polo during the time of Kublai Khan in the thirteenth century had a great impact on Europe.

Even so, the Chinese exerted little or no effort to share their cultural or spiritual knowledge with outsiders, a quality that contrasted directly with Christian, Buddhist and Muslim missionaries worldwide, who would inform and convert anyone they could to their religion.

Contact with China by Europeans was almost nonexistent even after they acquired the ability to circumnavigate the Horn of Africa. Then, in 1842, British gunboats forced China to open its doors for trade. However, Chinese was one of the most difficult languages to learn. Few Westerners who traveled to China were either sufficiently linguistically capable or interested enough to penetrate the culture and become knowledgeable insiders to authentic Chinese spiritual practices, especially Taoism. Consequently, most Chinese works on Taoism have yet to be adequately translated, even today.

Taoism: Lost in Translation

Although some Taoist texts have been translated into European or English languages, most notably the *Tao Te Ching* and *I Ching*, there are many issues with those translations. Few of the translators knew the original language well enough to understand the context behind the words they were translating or, worse, were not personally knowledgeable about the subjects they were translating. Using a dictionary of grammar and vocabulary to translate anything always carries with it the possibility of lacking context. Without context, meaning is easily lost or distorted. Nevertheless, anyone translating old texts or offering an analysis can write a book—even if they don't completely understand what they are writing about. When this occurred, more problems were caused downstream by other writers, who also didn't know the original language, and based their well-written (and possibly influential) works either partially or fully on the inaccurate context provided by the previous misleading translations. In this way confusion and distortion continued to be passed downstream.

To add to the confusion, some translators, who were familiar with Hinduism or Buddhism (at least in literary form), were unfamiliar with Taoist philosophy and therefore presented Taoist ideas in a muddled, imprecise way. Without realizing it, they substituted and interlaced Buddhist and Hindu perspectives when describing Taoism. This occurred because those translators could not see the Taoist works separately from the powerful imprint of their previous backgrounds in these other spiritual traditions.

Other translators, because they misunderstood the intent and relevance behind the words of Taoist sacred texts, simply created eloquent prose that rolled off the tongue easily but distorted the intent behind them. If they had any experiential knowledge of the practices themselves, it was minimal at best. This is akin to having heard of Jesus, but not having the faintest clue about how to pray or viewing Jesus primarily just as another variation of the Hindu god Krishna.

Renowned Scottish Victorian scholar James Legge was the first professor of Chinese at Oxford University (1876–1897). In association with Max Müller, he prepared the monumental and academic Sacred Books of the East series, published in fifty volumes between 1879 and 1891. Legge was a Scottish Congregationalist representative of the London Missionary Society in Malacca and Hong Kong (1840–1873). It would be questionable to consider him to be an insider of Eastern much less Taoist spiritual traditions. He most likely looked at the tradition though the lens of his Christian faith.

In the 1960s, during the explosion of Western interest in Eastern religions, came popular interest in the *I Ching*. The fundamental translation used was that of Richard Wilhelm, which in part gained acceptance because of his association with Carl Jung. Jung was a close protégé of psychologist Sigmund Freud, known for his work with psychological archetypes. Jung strongly influenced the transpersonal psychology movement.

The Wilhelm translation was written in the early twentieth century with the help of Taoist priests at Beijing's White Cloud Temple (Bai Yun Guan). This is the most important Taoist temple in North China (see p. 18). I spent a fair amount of time practicing sitting meditation there during the 1980s. In my discussions with Taoist priests at the temple, Wilhelm was well-remembered. They said that Wilhelm tried his best, but had insufficient background to completely understand the text from the Taoist perspective.

Thomas Cleary is the noted University of California (Berkeley) translator of the *Taoist I Ching* and many other Taoist texts. His books are well-written. However, to the best of my knowledge, he was not a practicing Taoist but rather a Buddhist, which in my opinion is reflected in his translations.

The Explosion of Interest in Indian Spiritual Traditions in the 1960s

The 1960s saw an increasing fascination with Eastern religions and philosophy. The Beatles visited Maharishi Mahesh Yogi in India. Numerous American, European and Australian hash-smoking hippies and comparative religion students and professors traveled to India and Nepal and became exposed to many gurus and forms of Hinduism and Buddhism. Many returned with their gurus or lamas, who then taught in the West. Books were written promoting the teachings of these gurus. More translations of classic scriptures appeared, continually improving in quality. This allowed the next round of India's spiritual knowledge to spread in the West.

What about Interest in Taoism?

In 1949, Mao Zedong's Communist Revolution established the People's Republic of China, closing off mainland China to the outside world. Only two small areas of China, Hong Kong and Taiwan, remained open to Westerners. Its spiritual knowledge—especially Taoism, which is uniquely Chinese—was essentially locked down tight.

It wasn't until the 1990s that travel to mainland China became relatively easy for European business people. Even at this point, few had the tenacity to crack the

Chinese language barrier sufficiently to seriously penetrate into Taoism. That is why the answer to the question, "What is Taoism?" still remains relatively hidden to the West. Cross-cultural transfer takes time, and the anxious, hurried mentality of modern life doesn't bode well for the clear transmission of many traditions.

From a comparative perspective, although knowledge about Chinese Buddhism traveled to India, Taoism didn't, so the Europeans lacked access to its teachings even from India's back door. Although Taoism could be found in Southeast Asia, the Chinese language barrier stopped most outsiders from understanding it. Even when English became more common between Indians and Europeans, the Chinese language remained almost completely impenetrable. That is why, until today, most texts and living spiritual teachers available in English-speaking nations are more focused on Indian Buddhism and its metamorphosis in China than on Taoism.

Today the situation is essentially unchanged. Access is dramatically greater in the West to India's spiritual knowledge rather than China's Taoism. It is more common for the leading spiritual lights of Hinduism and Buddhism to speak or write in English, or at least to have good translators, and many of them are willing to come to the West to teach. When China invaded Tibet and occupied it in 1949, Tibetan spiritual leaders fled and emigrated to India and other countries. It became essential for them to continue to grow and spread their spiritual knowledge, as well as to raise money for their monasteries in the new countries that took them in.

In contrast, it is rare for the leading lights of China's Taoism to either be willing to come to the West, to have studied English or to have satisfactory translators for their works.

APPENDIX C
The Energy Anatomy of the Body

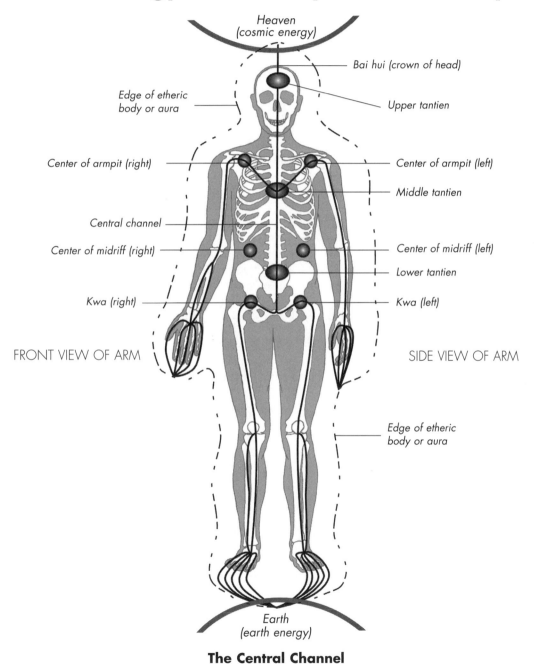

Heaven
(cosmic energy)

Bai hui (crown of head)

Edge of etheric
body or aura

Upper tantien

Center of armpit (right)

Center of armpit (left)

Middle tantien

Central channel

Center of midriff (right)

Center of midriff (left)

Lower tantien

Kwa (right)

Kwa (left)

FRONT VIEW OF ARM

SIDE VIEW OF ARM

Edge of etheric
body or aura

Earth
(earth energy)

The Central Channel

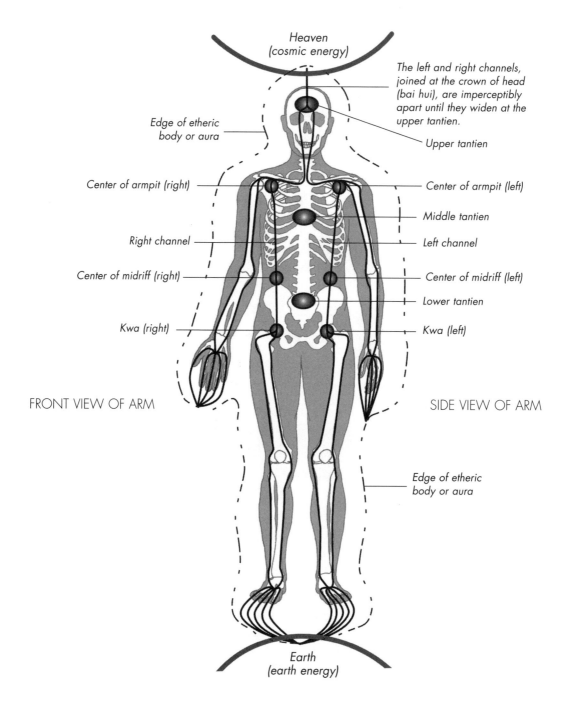

Heaven
(cosmic energy)

The left and right channels,
joined at the crown of head
(bai hui), are imperceptibly
apart until they widen at the
upper tantien.

Upper tantien

Edge of etheric
body or aura

Center of armpit (right)

Center of armpit (left)

Middle tantien

Right channel

Left channel

Center of midriff (right)

Center of midriff (left)

Lower tantien

Kwa (right)

Kwa (left)

FRONT VIEW OF ARM

SIDE VIEW OF ARM

Edge of etheric
body or aura

Earth
(earth energy)

The Left and Right Channels

APPENDIX D

Lineages and Training Chronology

The Author's Martial Arts Training

Martial Art	Location of Training	Dates of Training
Judo	New York; Tokyo	1961–67; 67–70
Karate	New York; Tokyo; Okinawa	1961–67; 67–69; 70
Jujitsu	New York	1962–66
Aikido	New York; Tokyo	1963–67; 67–69
Iaido	New York	1965–66
Cantonese White Crane	New York	1966–67
Monkey Boxing	New York	1966–67
Bagua	Tokyo/Taiwan Taiwan/Hong Kong Beijing	1968–71 1974–75, 77–79, 83, 87, 89 1981, 83–86
Tai Chi	Tokyo/Taiwan Hong Kong/Taiwan Xiamen Beijing	1968–71 1974–75, 77–79, 83, 87, 89, 97 1983–84 1981, 83–86
Hsing-i	Tokyo/Taiwan Hong Kong/Taiwan Beijing	1968–71 1974–75, 77–79,83, 87, 89 1981, 83–86
Fukien White Crane	Tokyo; Taiwan	1971; 74–75
Wing Chun	New York; Hong Kong	1972, 76; 74, 75, 77
Chinese Wrestling	Taiwan	1974
Northern Monkey Boxing	Taiwan	1974–75, 78
Eight Drunken Immortals	Taiwan	1974–75, 78
Praying Mantis	Taiwan	1974–75
Northern Shaolin	Hong Kong	1983

Note: At the time of these trainings, traditional Chinese teachers of the internal martial arts usually did not issue certificates to students. However, certain documentation was presented to the author, some of which appears in the following sections. The above chart does not include the author's training in the related arts of meditation, qigong, tui na and other bodywork disciplines, nor does it cover his two years in India studying yoga, kundalini and tantra.

Lineages

This lineage information was provided to Bruce Kumar Frantzis by Liu Hung Chieh. Liu said that it was not possible to list all the lineage masters. In Liu's words, "The masters listed here are the important ones, and their art is handed down directly by the Old Generation."

The Chinese names bestowed on me as a lineage holder were Fan Quingren (literary name) and Fan Zhishan (spoken or ordinary name).

Bagua Lineage

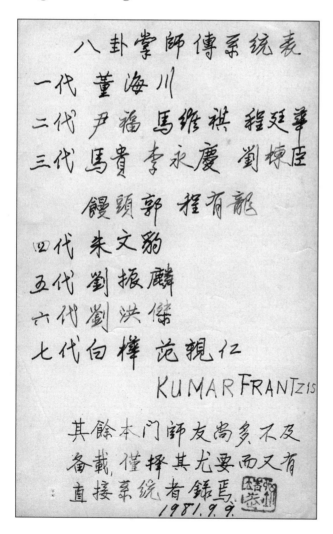

The Name List of Bagua Masters

The First Generation:
Tung Hai Chuan

The Second Generation:
Yin Fu
Ma Weiqi
Cheng Ting Hua

The Third Generation:
Ma Gui
Li Yongqing
Liu Jianchen
Mantou Guo

The Fourth Generation:
Zhu Wenbao

The Fifth Generatiion:
Liu Zhenlin

The Sixth Generatiion:
Liu Hung Chieh

The Seventh Generation:
Bai Hua
Fan Qingren (Kumar Frantzis)

Tai Chi Lineage

The Name List of Tai Chi Masters

Chang San Feng (A legendary Taoist figure)

↓

Wang Tsung Yueh

↓

Chen Wang Ting

↓

Chen Hsing

↓

Yang Lu Chan

↓   ↘

Yang Pan Hou   Chuan You

↓   ↙

Wu Jien Chuan

↓

Liu Hung Chieh

↓

Fan Qingren (Kumar Frantzis)

Hsing-i Lineage

**The Name List of Hsing-i Masters
(Since Li Luo Neng, Shen County,
Hebei Province)**

1. Li Luo Neng

2. Liu Qilan,   Guo Yun Shen

3. Li Tsung I,   Chang Chao-Tung,   Li Kuiyuan

4. Li Yunshan,   Shang Yunxiang,   Sun Lu Tang

5. Li Jianqiu,   Jin Yunding

6. Liu Hung Chieh

7. Bai Hua,   Fan Qingren (Kumar Frantzis)

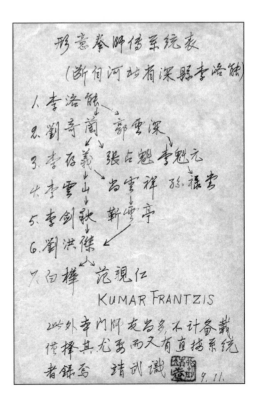

Certificates

Bagua

KUMAR FRANTZIS 賜名"范親仁"字
"志善"為吾八卦门中傑出之弟子功夫純
熟身手矯健今夏來華親受庭訓能舉一
反三心領神會勤學苦練虛心請益盡鮮
其區誠所謂好之者不如樂之者也茲將
返美特乞一言以為贈用書數語以為勖
焉

　　　劉 洪傑 靖武 誌於北京州
　　舍 [印]
　　　1981.9.6日
　　辛酉年八月初九日

(Bruce) Kumar Frantzis, whose bestowed names are Fan Qingren and Fan Zhishan, is an outstanding disciple of our bagua *men* (tradition). His art is highly skilled, and his body and hands are strong and vigorous.

This summer Kumar Frantzis came to China and was personally trained in our courtyard. He is able to draw inferences about other cases from one instance, to understand tacitly and to study diligently and train hard. He is open-minded and is good at learning from others. Few people in the world can match him. It is said that people who are professional are not as good as people who really enjoy what they are doing.

Upon his returning to the United States, it is my honor to write a few words to praise and encourage him.

Liu Hongjie (Liu Hung Chieh)
In teaching courtyard, Beijing, September 11, 1981

Tai Chi

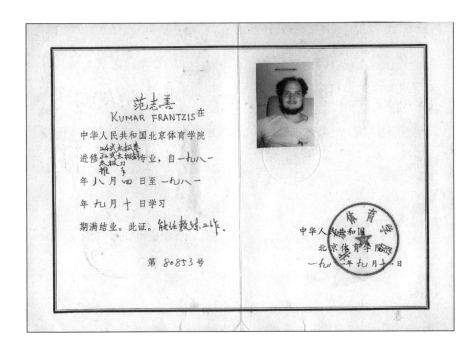

(Bruce) Kumar Frantzis completed his further studies of tai chi chuan in 24 patterns, tai chi sword in 32 patterns, tai chi knife and Tui Shou (Push Hands) at Beijing Institute of Physical Education, Beijing, People's Republic of China, from August 4, 1981 to September 10, 1981. He is qualified to be a coach.

Beijing Institute of Physical Education
Beijing
People's Republic of China

Certificate No. 80853
September 11, 1981

Hsing-i

KUMAR FRANTZIS 賜名范親仁字志善為吾
形意門中傑出之弟子功夫純熟身手矯健今夏來
華親受庭訓能舉一反三心領神會勤學苦練虛心
請益大有一日千里之勢余深喜之誠屬不世出之奇
才也茲將返美特乞一言以為贈用書數語以為嘉勉
焉

劉　洪傑　靖武　📷
📷誌於北京艸堂

1981. 9. 11.
辛酉年八月十四日

(Bruce) Kumar Frantzis, whose bestowed names are Fan Qingren and Fan Zhishan, is an outstanding disciple of our hsing-i *men* (tradition). His gung fu (skill) is very good, and his movements are quick and perfect.

This summer he came to China and I personally trained him. When I tell him "A," he already knows "Z." He understands everything from his heart and soul. He is diligent and practices hard. He is very humble when he asks questions. In one day of practice he can go a thousand miles. I am very happy that he is a very special and outstanding student.

Upon his returning to the United States, it is my honor to write a few words to praise and encourage him.

Liu Hongjie (Liu Hung Chieh)
In teaching courtyard, Beijing, September 11, 1981

APPENDIX E

Transliterations and Meanings of Chinese Terms

Pinyin	Yale	Wade Giles	Chinese Traditional	Simplified	English
An	An	An	按	按	"Press down," any downward-moving energy or power
Bagua/ba gua	Ba gwa	Pa kua	八卦	八卦	Bagua
Bagua men	Ba gwa men	Pa kua men	八卦門	八卦门	"Bagua door," a bagua school that retains the full martial tradition
Bagua zhang	Ba gwa jang	Pa kua chang	八卦掌	八卦掌	Bagua zhang
Ba mu zhang	Ba mu jang	Pa mu chang	八母掌	八母掌	Eight Mother Palms
Bai bu	Bai bu	Pai pu	擺步	摆步	Toe-out step
Bai hui	Bai hwei	Pai hui	百會	百会	"Hundred meetings," crown energy gate
Bai shi	Bai shr	Pai shih	拜師	拜师	Disciple
Bian hua	Byan hwa	Pien hua	變化	变化	Change
Bu	Bu	Pu	步	步	Step
Cai	Tsai	Ts'ai	採	采	Pluck or pull down
Chan si jin	Chan sz jin	Ch'an szu chin	纏絲勁	缠丝劲	The silk-coiling technique of Chen style tai chi chuan, wherein the soft tissues of the body twist and turn dramatically
Chang	Chang	Ch'ang	長	长	Length(en), long
Chang quan	Chang chywan	Ch'ang ch'üan	長拳	长拳	Long fist, the basic method of Northern Shaolin external martial arts
Chou si jin	Chou sz jin	Ch'ou szu chin	抽絲勁	抽丝劲	Pulling silk power
Da Cheng Quan	Da Cheng Chywan	Ta Ch'eng Ch'üan	大成拳	大成拳	Another name for Yi Chuan
Dao	Dau	Tao	道	道	Way
Dao de	Dau de	Tao te	道德	道德	Spiritual morality
Dao jia	Dau jya	Tao chia	道家	道家	Philosophical Taoism
Dao jiao	Dau jyau	Tao chiao	道教	道教	Religious Taoism
Dan huan zhang	Dan hwan jang	Tan huan chang	單換掌	单换掌	Single palm change
Dantian/dan tian	Dan tyan	Tan t'ien	丹田	丹田	The three primary centers in the human body where chi collects, disperses and recirculates. They govern the energetic anatomy of a person. The practices of the three tantiens are at the operational root of all Chinese chi practices.
De	De	Te	德	德	Virtue, power
Deng jiao	Deng jyau	Teng chiao	蹬腳	蹬脚	Step the heel/foot; push heel back; heel kick
Di ban gong fu	Di ban gung fu	Ti pan kung fu	底半功夫	底半功夫	"Lower half gong fu," skill of the lower body
Dui	Dwei	Tui	兌	兑	Joy (Gua)

Pinyin	Yale	Wade Giles	Chinese Traditional	Simplified	English
Dui shou	Dwei shou	Tui shou	對手	对手	Palm(s) face(s) you
Fa qi	Fa chi	Fa ch'i	發氣	发气	Release/emit energy
Fa jin	Fa jin	Fa chin	發勁	发劲	Release/emit power
Fan shou	Fan shou	Fan shou	翻手	翻手	Palm(s) turn(s) away from you
Feng shui	Feng shwei	Feng shui	風水	风水	Feng shui, geomancy
Gen	Gen	Ken	艮	艮	Mountain (Gua)
Gong fu	Gung fu	Kung fu	功夫	功夫	(i) Level of skill gained through long, continuous effort in anything
					(ii) Generic term for Chinese martial arts
Gua	Gwa	Kua	卦	卦	Trigram or hexagram
Hou Tian	Hou tyan	Hou T'ien	後天	后天	"After heaven," that which happens to a person after leaving the womb. Talents, skills, or accomplishments acquired after birth.
Ji	Ji	Chi	擠	擠	"Project forward," any energy that presses or projects in a forward direction
Ji ben gong	Ji ben gung	Chi pen kung	基本功	基本功	Basic power training
Jin	Jin	Chin	勁	劲	Power
Jing	Jing	Ching	精	精	Sperm, essence, body
Jing	Jing	Ching	靜	静	Still(ness), calm, quiet
Jing luo	Jing lwo	Ching lo	經絡	经络	Acupuncture meridian
Kai he	Kai he	K'ai he	開合	开合	"Open-close," the universal pulsing that occurs at the subatomic level, cellular level and cosmological level
Kou tou	Kou tou	K'ou t'ou	叩頭	叩头	Kowtow
Kou bu	Kou bu	K'ou pu	釦步	扣步	"Button step," toe-in step
Kua	Kwa	K'ua	胯	胯	Groin, inguinal area
Kan	Kan	K'an	坎	坎	Water (Gua)
Kun	Kwen	K'un	坤	坤	Earth (Gua)
Lao gong	Lau gung	Lao kung	勞宮	劳宫	Center of palm energy gate
Li	Li	Li	離	離	Fire (Gua)
Lie	lye	Lieh	挒	挒	Split
Liang yi	Lyang yi	Liang I	兩儀	两仪	The two powers (yin and yang)
Liu he	lyou he	Liu he	六合	六合	The six harmonies/combinations
Liu he ba fa	lyou he ba fa	Liu he pa fa	六合八法	六合八法	"Six harmonies, eight methods," a completely internal Chinese martial art
Luo xuan jin	Luo sywan jin	Luo hsüan chin	螺旋勁	螺旋劲	Drilling power
Lu	Lu	Lu	将	捋	The absorbing, yielding energy of the internal martial arts. This term is especially used in tai chi chuan.
Mingmen/ming men	Ming men	Ming men	命門	命门	Life door

Pinyin	Yale	Wade Giles	Chinese Traditional	Simplified	English
Nei	Nei	Nei	內	内	Inside/internal
Nei ba zhang	Nei ba jang	Nei pa chang	內八掌	内八掌	Inner eight palms
Nei chan	Nei chan	Nei ch'an	內纏	内缠	Inward twisting (Chen style)
Nei dan	Nei dan	Nei tan	內丹	内丹	Internal alchemy
Neigong/nei gong	Nei gung	Nei kung	內功	内功	Internal work. The original chi cultivation system in China invented by the Taoists.
Nei jia	Nei jya	Nei chia	內家	内家	All the Taoist energy practices described as one family
Nei jia quan	Nei chywan	Nei chia ch'üan	內家拳	内家拳	All the internal martial arts described as one family
Nei jin	Nei jin	Nei chin	內勁	内劲	Internal power
Nei san he	Nei san he	Nei san he	內三合	内三合	Internal three harmonies/combinations. The three internal components of the mind in Taoist theory: the yi, chi and shen, which must be united in Chinese internal martial arts practices.
Peng	Peng	P'eng	掤	掤	"Expanding," the rising, pushing-outward internal power that forms the basis of the yang chi aspect of internal martial arts
Qi	Chi	Ch'i	氣	气	Energy, subtle life force, internal energy, internal power. Manifested energy that empowers something to work and function.
Qi chu zuo	Chi chu dzwo	Ch'i ch'u tso	氣出做	气出做	The direct movement of chi by the heart-mind
Qigong/qi gong	Chi gung	Ch'i kung	氣功	气功	Energy work, the ancient Chinese art and science of developing and cultivating chi by one's own effort
Qigong tui na	Chi gung twei na	Ch'i kung t'ui na	氣功推拿	气功推拿	Therapeutic bodywork with chi
Qi jing ba mai	Chi jing ba mai	Ch'i ching pa mai	奇經八脈	奇经八脉	The eight extraordinary meridians of acupuncture
Qian	Chyan	Ch'ien	乾	乾	Heaven (Gua)
Qin na	Chin na	Ch'in na	擒拿	擒拿	"Seizing the joints," the branch of Chinese martial arts concerned with using joint-locks and used to pull, rip or tear skin by grabbing
Quan	Chywan	Ch'üan	拳	拳	"Fist," fighting art
Rou shou	Rou shou	Jou shou	柔手	柔手	Soft Hands, also known as San Shou or Free Hands in Taiwan. A two-person fighting preparation technique practiced in bagua (and some hsing-i schools) in which the arms of the partners are in continuous spiraling contact.
San jiao	San jyau	San chiao	三膲	三焦	Triple burner (Three burners)
San ti	San ti	San t'i	三体	三体	The primary hsing-i standing posture
Shaolin gong fu	Shaulin gung fu	Shaolin kung fu	少林功夫	少林功夫	Shaolin gong fu, the external martial art associated with the Shaolin Monastery in Henan Province, China
Shen	Shen	Shen	神	神	Spirit or consciousness
Shi da tian gang	Shr da tyan gang	Shih ta, t'ien kang	十大天干	十大天干	Ten heavenly stems
Shun shi zhang	Shwun shr jang	Shun shih chang	順勢掌	顺势掌	Smooth palm change
Taiji	Taiji	T'ai chi	太極	太极	Philosophical term indicating the non-dual origin of yin and yang

Pinyin	Yale	Wade Giles	Chinese Traditional	Simplified	English
Taijiquan / taiji quan	Taiji chywan	T'ai chi ch'üan	太極拳	大极拳	"Supreme ultimate martial arts fist." One of the three internal martial arts of China, most known for its emphasis on softness, slow-motion movement, and its sophisticated qigong methodology based on whole-body physical coordination.
Tang ni bu	Tang ni bu	T'ang ni pu	趟泥步	趟泥步	Mud walking
Ting jin	Ting jin	T'ing chin	聽勁	听劲	Listening power
Tui na	Twei na	T'ui na	推拿	推拿	Therapeutic bodywork
Tui shou	Twei shou	T'ui shou	推手	推手	Push Hands
Wai ba zhang	Wai ba jang	Wai pa chang	外八掌	外八掌	External eight palms
Wai chan	Wai chan	Wai ch'an	外纏	外缠	Outward twisting (Chen style)
Wai jia	Wai jya	Wai chia	外家	外家	The external martial arts described as one family
Wai jia quan	Wai jya chywan	Wai chia ch'üan	外家拳	外家拳	The external martial arts described as one family
Wei qi	Wei chi	Wei ch'i	衛氣	卫气	Protective chi. The layer of energy between a person's skin and muscle that protects against disease entering the body from the external environment.
Wu	Wu	Wu	無	无	Nothing, Emptiness
Wu ji	Wu ji	Wu chi	無極	无极	The not-ultimate (the source of Taiji)
Wu wei from	Wu wei	Wu wei	無為	无为	"Doing without doing," the fundamental Taoist concept of having action arise an empty mind without preconception or agenda, action that operates by simply following the natural course of universal energy as it manifests itself without strain or ego involvement
Wushu	Wushu	Wushu	武術	武术	A generic term for martial arts in China
Xian tian	Syan tyan	Hsien t'ien	先天	先天	"Before heaven," whatever has happened to a human between conception and the time of birth
Xin	Syin	Hsin	心	心	"Heart-mind," the ultimate source of a person's being according to classical Taoist and Buddhist thought. The hsin is both subtle and nonphysical and is located near the physical heart.
Xing	Sying	Hsing	形	形	Form
Xing yi quan	Sying yi chywan	Hsing-i ch'üan	形意拳	形意拳	Mind-form boxing. A hard internal martial art created by the Chinese general Yue Fei in the thirteenth century. Hsing-i emphasizes all aspects of the mind to create its forms and fighting movements.
Xun	Syun	Hsün	巽	巽	Compliance (Gua)
Yang	Yang	Yang	陽	阳	Yang
Yi	Yi	I	意	意	Intent
Yi chu zuo	Yi chu dzwo	I ch'u tso	意出做	意出做	Intention moves the chi
Yiquan	Yi chywan	I ch'üan	形意拳	形意拳	A style of hsing-i that is based upon eight standing postures rather than on the classical movements of hsing-i. Yiquan was developed by combining classical hsing-i with bagua footwork, Western boxing and Buddhist qigong.

Pinyin	Yale	Wade Giles	Chinese Traditional	Simplified	English
Yin	Yin	Yin	陰	阴	Yin
Yong fa	Yung fa	Yung fa	用法	用法	Fighting applications
Zhan zhuang	Jan jwang	Chan chuang	站樁	站	"Standing like a post," standing in postures. Used to develop internal power and connection
Zhen	Jen	Chen	震	震	Thunder/Quake (Gua)
Zheng qi	Jeng chi	Cheng ch'i	真氣	真气	Genuine chi or unifying chi. The one chi that unifies all the chi of the body which all Taoist internal arts seek to cultivate
Zhong mai	Jung mai	Chung mai	沖脈	冲脉	Central channel
Zhuan jin	Jwan jin	Chuan chin	轉勁	转劲	Twisting power
Zi ran	Dz ran	Tzu jan	自然	自然	Nature/natural

PROPER NAMES

Pinyin	Yale	Wade Giles	Chinese Traditional	Simplified
Bai Hua	Bai Pai	Hua Pai	白樺	白桦
Chen	Chen	Ch'en	陳	陈
Cheng Tinghua	Cheng Ting Hwa	Ch'eng T'ing Hua	程廷華	程廷华
Daodejing	Daudejing	Tao Te Ching	道德經	道德经
Dao Zang	Dau Zang	Tao Tsang	道藏	道藏
Dong Hai Chuan	Dung Hai Chwan	Tung Hai Ch'uan	董海川	董海川
Fan Qingren	Fan Chingren	Fan Ch'ing Jen	范親仁	范亲仁
Gao Yi Sheng	Gau Yi Sheng	Kao I Sheng	高義盛	高义盛
Hao	Hau	Hao	郝	郝
Hong Yi Xiang	Hung Yi Syang	Hung I Hsiang	洪懿祥	洪懿祥
Li Feng Chun	Li Feng Chwun	Li Feng Ch'un	劉鳳春	刘凤春
Laozi	Laudz	Lao Tzu	老子	老子
Liu Hong Jie	Lyou Hung Jye	Liu Hung Chieh	劉洪傑	刘洪杰
Luo De Xiu	Lwo De Syou	Lo Te-Hsiu	羅德修	罗德修
Ma Gui	Ma Gwei	Ma Kui	馬貴	马贵
Ma Shi Qing	Ma Shr Ching	Ma Shih Ch'ing	馬世卿	馬世卿
Ma Weiqi	Ma Weichi	Ma Weich'i	馬維棋	馬維棋
Ong Shen Ming				
Song Chang Rong	Sung Chang Rung	Sung Ch'ang Jung	宋長榮	宋长荣
Tianjin	Tyanjin	T'ien Chin	天津	天津

PROPER NAMES, CONT.

Pinyin	Yale	Wade Giles	Chinese Traditional	Simplified	English
Wang Shu Jin	Wang Shu Jin	Wang Shu Chin	王樹金	王树金	
Wang Xiang Zhai	Wang Syang Jai	Wang Hsiang Chai	王薌齋	王薌斋	
Wu	Wu	Wu	武	武	
Wu	Wu	Wu	吳	吴	
Wu Jian Quan	Wu Jyan Chywan	Wu Chien-ch'uan	吳鑑泉	吳鑑泉	
Wu Yuxiang	Wu Yusyang	Wu Yü Hsiang	武禹襄	武禹襄	
Yang	Yang	Yang	楊	楊	
Yang Cheng Fu	Yang Cheng Fu	Yang Ch'eng Fu	楊澄甫	楊澄甫	
Yin Fu	Yin Fu	Yin Fu	尹福	尹福	
Yijing	Yijing	I Ching	易經	易经	
Zhuangzi	Jwangdz	Chuang Tzu	莊子	莊子	

PHRASES

Pinyin	Yale	Wade Giles	Chinese Traditional	Simplified	English
Bu diu bu ding	Bu dyou bu ding	Pu fiu pu ting	不丟不頂	不丢不顶	Neither leave nor oppose
Han xiong ba bei	Han syung ba bei	Han hsiung pa pei	涵胸拔	涵胸拔背	Chest relaxes down, back rises
Shi fu jin men	Shi fu jin men	Shi fu jin men	師傅進門	师傅进门	The teacher takes you into the gate,
Lian zai ge xin	Lyan dzai ge syin	Lien tsai ke hsin	練在各心	练在各心	The practice is yours and is from the heart
Liu tun shou kua	Lyou twun shou kwa	Liu t'un shou k'ua	溜臀收胯	溜臀收胯	Buttocks forward and shrink the kwa
Tong ze bu teng	Tung dze bu teng	T'ung tse pu t'eng	通則不疼	通则不疼	Flow then no pain
Teng ze bu tong	Teng dze bu tung	T'eng tse pu t'ung	疼則不通	疼则不通	Pain then no flow
Wang Wo	Wang Wo	Wang Wo	忘我	忘我	Forget yourself
Wei lu zhong zheng	Wei lu jung jeng	Wei lu chung cheng	尾閭中正	尾闾中正	Tailbone centrally aligned
Wei lu xiang qian	Wei lu syang chyan	Wei lu hsiang ch'ien	尾閭向前	尾闾向前	Tailbone forward
Zou huo ru mo	Dzou hwo ru mwo	Tsou huo ju mo	走火入魔	走火入魔	"Fire goes to the devil." This is a metaphor for problems caused by practicing incorrect forceful qigong techniques.

Table compiled by Matthew Brewer

APPENDIX F

Glossary

A

Aikido A Japanese internal energy-based martial art created by Morihei Ueshiba in the 1930s.

Application The practical use or range of uses of a particular technique in the martial arts, Chinese medicine or meditation.

Aura The energetic or bioelectric field that surrounds the living human body. *See also* Etheric body.

B

Bagua/bagua zhang (bagua/bagua chang, pakua chang, bagwa jang) Eight trigram palm bagua is one of China's three main internal martial arts. It is a Taoist practice based on the *I Ching,* which is simultaneously a longevity practice, a martial art, a healing modality, and a spiritual/meditation practice.

Bagua qigong postures The practice in which an individual holds his or her arms motionless in space, whether or not the feet are moving. The practice is done in order to bring the chi from the belly and spine to the fingertips and stabilize the internal ligaments of the upper body.

Bien hua (pien hua, bian hua) To change; changes. The nature of change itself. Basic to Taoism and the *I Ching* is that everything in the phenomenal universe is in the process of changing, except the Tao, which remains changeless. What occurs during the shift, how the change transpires, and the final result of the change are all aspects of bien hua. The term also applies to the shift experienced during Taoist alchemy between one level of energy or consciousness and another level, either higher or lower. Refers also to the way you change from one fighting technique to another technique in internal martial arts or from one healing intervention to another in qigong tui na.

Buddhism One of the world's major religions. Buddhism is based on the meditation teachings of Gautama the Buddha who lived and taught in India in the sixth century B.C. Buddhism has mostly vanished from India since the Muslim invasions occurring from the thirteenth to the sixteenth century, and is most prevalent in the cultures of Oriental Asia—China, Japan, Korea, Southeast Asia, and Tibet.

C

Central channel (zhong mai, chung mai, jung mai) The main energy channel located in the exact center of the human body between the perineum and the crown of the head and extending through the bone marrow of the arms and legs.

Chan sz jin (chan si jin) The silk-coiling technique of Chen style tai chi chuan, wherein the soft tissues of the body twist and turn dramatically.

Chen village tai chi The original form of tai chi chuan.

Chi (qi, ch'i; ki in Japanese) Energy, subtle life force, internal energy, internal power. Manifested energy that empowers something to work and function. This concept underlies Chinese, Japanese, and Korean culture, in which the world is perceived not purely in terms of physical matter, but also in terms of invisible energy.

Chi chu dzuo (qi chu zuo, ch'i ch'u tso) The method of moving a felt bodily sensation of chi as a live force from the lower tantien into whichever energy channels the practitioner consciously directs it.

Chinese calligraphy A method of writing Chinese characters or symbolic concepts with pictures using a brush and ink. Calligraphy is considered by the Chinese to be a high form of fine art and a form of intellectual qigong, one of its distinguishing characteristics being that chi, or energy, is projected onto the written surface.

Chinese medicine (TCM) The 3000-year-old traditional medical system of China. Its basic branches are acupuncture, bonesetting, qigong, qigong na, herbalism, and moxibustion. Its therapeutic interventions are not based so much on regulating the physical matter of the body but rather on regulating the subtle energy (chi), which tells the matter how to behave.

Circle Walking The primary training method of the internal martial art of bagua.

Combination Form tai chi A form wherein one or several styles of tai chi and/or hsing-i, bagua or Shaolin are mixed together within a single form.

D

Dissolving process A neigong technique for releasing bound energy both from within the human body and the etheric body.

Double Palm Change A movement that is the basis of all the yin, soft, or amorphous techniques of bagua zhang.

E

Earth Element In Chinese cosmology, one of the basic energies or elements from which all manifested phenomena are created.

Eight energetic bodies In Taoist philosophy, eight clear vibratory frequencies of energy that comprise a human being. Each is called a "body." These are identified as the physical body, etheric/chi body or aura, emotional body, mental body, psychic energy body, causal/karmic body, body of individuality or essence, and body of the Tao.

Eight Mother Palms (ba mu chang, ba mu zhang, pa mu chang, ba mu jang) The eight basic palm changes or movement patterns of bagua zhang. Each of the energies of the eight trigrams of the *I Ching* is embodied in one of the Eight Mother Palms.

Emptiness A profound state of spiritual, mental and psychic equilibrium that is a major goal of all Asian meditation practices and that lies at the heart of the higher levels of achievement in the internal martial arts.

Energy channels of the body All the subtle energetic channels of the body through which chi travels.

Etheric body (chi body) The bioelectric field that extends anywhere from a few inches to a few hundred feet from a person's body. Commonly called the aura in the West.

External/internal martial arts (nei wai quan/chuan) Those martial arts that use both a clearly developed internal qigong program and external muscular practices based on contracting the muscles through physical tension.

External martial arts (wai jia quan, wai chia ch'uan) Martial arts that focus on physicality, muscular strength, reflexes, tension, mental discipline, and body conditioning (push-ups, sit-ups, weight-lifting, and running), and not on developing and cultivating chi.

F

Feng shui The mathematical occult science of Chinese geomancy where one locates the energy lines, relationships, and points of a physical site on the earth. The site could be a piece of land, a building, or arrangements of the objects within a room. The chi of the site is then analyzed to determine its positive or negative effects on manifesting wealth, love relationships, family harmony, spirituality or on whether certain types of events will be successful or not. Techniques can then be employed to mitigate bad fortune or enhance good fortune.

Fighting application The practical use or range of uses for combat of a specific technique of a martial art.

Fire Element In Chinese cosmology, one of the basic energies or elements from which all manifested phenomena are created.

Fire method A meditation or energetic technique that emphasizes pushing your limits and using full effort to 100 percent of your capacities.

Frame The physical shape and energetic qualities that an internal martial arts posture assumes, ranging from small and condensed (small frame) to large and expansive (large frame).

H

Hao style tai chi The least widespread style of tai chi; based on small external and internal movements.

Hexagram One of the sixty-four energetic changes of the *I Ching.*

Hinduism A major religion of India that reaches as far back as recorded time. Its most important texts are the Vedas, Upanishads, and the Bhagavad Gita. Hinduism gave birth to Yoga, Tantra, and Buddhism.

Hsin (xin, shin) Heart-Mind. The ultimate source of a person's being according to classical Taoist and Buddhist thought. The hsin is both subtle and nonphysical, and is located near the physical heart.

Hsing-i/hsing-i chuan (xing yi/xingyi quan, shing yi chuan) Mind-form boxing. A hard internal martial art created by Chinese general Yue Fei in the thirteenth century. Hsing-i emphasizes all aspects of the mind to create its forms and fighting movements.

I

I (yi) Will, intent, intention, mind, and projecting mind. In the chi world of China, "I" (pronounced yee) denotes the specific aspect of mind that projects. If a person sees something and wants to acquire or move toward the object of his or her intention (be it concrete or mental), that person mobilizes the "I," and after an infinitesimal gap moves into action.

I Ching (yi jing) *Book of Changes.* This 5,000-year-old book is considered to be the classic Taoist text about the nature of change and how change occurs. The *I Ching* encompasses eight trigrams that embody the eight primal chi energies of which the universe is composed, according to Taoist thought. The eight expand to sixty-four by detailing how each of the individual trigrams impacts, mitigates, and expands the others when they are mixed. Bagua zhang is a mind/body/spirit practice that seeks to have an individual experience within his or her own being what the *I Ching* communicates intellectually.

I Chuan (yiquan) Also known as Da Cheng Chuan. A style of hsing-i that is based upon eight standing postures rather than on the classical movements of hsing-i. I Chuan was developed by combining classical hsing-i with bagua footwork, Western boxing and Buddhist qigong.

I chu dzuo (yi chu zuo, i ch'u tso) A basic chi cultivation method where one uses the "I" to create a mental picture (visualization), which then indirectly moves chi through the human body according to the classic Chinese principle: The "I" leads or moves the chi.

Inner Dissolving process A basic Taoist chi (neigong) practice for releasing energy blocked anywhere within a person; used primarily to heal and strengthen an individual's emotional, mental and psychic aspects.

Internal alchemy (nei dan) The transformation, through meditation and certain mind/body/spirit practices, of an individual's inner energies for realizing and becoming one with the Tao, the nature of the universe itself.

Internal arts (nei jia, nei chia) Those energy arts in China that are concerned with cultivating meditation, the internal chi, and the inner aspects of a person's being rather than only his or her quantifiable external manifestations in the physical world.

Internal martial arts (nei jia quan/neijiaquan, nei chia ch'uan) Those fighting systems that base their power on cultivating chi, the mind, total relaxation, longevity and meditation rather than the purely physical means of the external martial arts. Although there are internal aspects to some of the external Shaolin martial arts, in China the term "internal martial arts" usually refers to the three Taoist martial arts of tai chi chuan, hsing-i chuan and bagua zhang.

J

Ji In the internal martial arts, any energy that presses or projects in a forward direction.

Ji ben gong (ji ben gung, chi ben kung) The basic power training through which all the Chinese martial arts develop the type of power they specialize in.

Jin (jing) Power.

Jing luo Collateral meridians. The acupuncture meridians that horizontally wrap around the body and connect its vertical acupuncture lines.

Judo A Japanese external martial art based on wrestling, joint-locks, submission holds and chokes. A descendant of the Chinese martial art of shuai jiao and the Japanese martial art of jujitsu. Judo has been an Olympic sport since the 1960s.

Jujitsu The unarmed combat external martial art of the samurai during Japan's feudal period. Based primarily on throws, joint-locks, submission holds, and chokes, with punches, kicks, and strikes being secondary.

K

Kai-he Opening and closing.

Karate The Japanese external martial art based primarily on kicks, punches, hand strikes, foot sweeps, and a few throws. Karate is primarily an empty-handed martial art, with limited weapons training.

Ki *See* Chi.

Kundalini A meditation method of India that uses energy work to unravel the mysteries of human consciousness and enlightenment.

Kung fu family (gung fu/gong fu family) A Chinese surrogate family structure based on martial arts or meditation. The teacher symbolizes the father, the students become the children, the people who studied earlier become older brothers/ sisters, new arrivals are younger brothers/sisters, and so forth.

Kwa (kua) The area on each side of the body extending from the inguinal ligaments through the inside of the pelvis to the top (crest) of the hip bones.

L

Lao gong (lao gung/kung) The energetic point in the center of the palm; the easiest point in the body from which to project chi externally.

Left channel One of the three primary energy lines in the body (on its left side), the other two being the right channel (its paired opposite), and the central channel. The paired opposites of the left and right channels of subtle energy are responsible for all the yin-yang dualistic functions of a human being, including the functioning of the body, emotions, psychic activity, and the manifestation of events in the outer world.

Liang yi (liang i) The interplay of yin and yang.

Lineage In the martial arts, an unbroken line of teaching that runs from one master through successive generations of worthy students, who become masters in their own right and pass on the knowledge.

Lineage disciple A formal disciple who is chosen to learn and carry forth to future generations all the intact knowledge of any specific lineage in such subjects as martial arts, meditation or qigong.

Lower tantien (dantian) Located below the navel in the center of the body, this energetic center is primarily responsible for the health of the human body. It is the only energy center where all the energy channels that affect the physical body intersect.

M

Martial arts Various fighting methodologies, both empty-handed and with weapons, that are concerned with formalized techniques of injuring or killing an attacker in the most efficient manner with the least harm to oneself.

Meditative stillness A level of accomplishment in meditation where the practitioner's mind becomes exceptionally quiet and rests relaxed and centered within itself.

Metal Element In Chinese cosmology, one of the basic energies or elements from which all manifested phenomena are created.

Middle burner Located in the torso between the solar plexus and the lower tantien. The energy that exists in this middle area of the body coordinates and harmonizes the chi of the upper and lower burners, which lie above and below the middle burner.

Middle tantien (dantian) One of the three major energy centers in the body. Two separate places are considered to be the middle tantien. They are located near each other, each governing different energetic functions. The point located at the solar plexus just below the sternum is responsible for the physical functions of the middle internal organs of the body (liver, spleen, and kidneys), as well as the will to persevere. The point located near the heart on the central channel governs physical, emotional, mental, psychic or causal relationships.

Moving meditation Any method of meditation wherein a practitioner is able to actualize the goals of meditation (including stilling the mind) while the body is in continuous motion.

N

Nei ba zhang The eight palms of bagua that are designed to put an individual in direct contact with the living energies upon which the eight trigrams of the *I Ching* are based.

Neigong (nei gung/kung) Internal power. The original chi cultivation (qigong) system in China invented by the Taoists. The Taoist neigong system forms the basis for the internal martial arts of bagua zhang, tai chi chuan and hsing-i chuan.

Nei jia Describes all the internal martial arts or Taoist chi practices as one family.

Nei jin (nei jing, nei chin) Internal power. A specific form of chi that integrates all the various energies of the body into one unified chi that can manifest physical power.

Nei san he The three internal components of the mind in Taoist theory: the "I" (intention), chi (energy) and shen (spirit or consciousness), all of which must be united in Chinese internal martial arts practices.

O

Open-close (kai-he) The Chinese yin-yang paired opposites concept of growing/ shrinking, expanding/contracting and lengthening/shortening, etc. This universal pulsing occurs at the subatomic, cellular and cosmological levels.

Outer Dissolving process A basic Taoist chi (neigong) practice for releasing blocked internal energy within the body and projecting it externally. Used primarily to heal and strengthen the energies related to the physical body.

P

Post-birth bagua The linear as opposed to Circle Walking practice of bagua zhang.

Post-birth chi The chi a human gets by eating, drinking, sleeping, breathing, and exercising.

Posture The last static position that ends a martial art technique or qigong movement. Also, a whole movement for which a specific martial art or qigong technique is named.

Pre-birth bagua The Circle-Walking practice of bagua whose purpose is to develop pre-birth chi in the same manner as it was done in Taoist monasteries.

Push Hands (tui shou) The continuous two-person hand-touching practice of the internal martial art of tai chi chuan, which forms the bridge between the form movements of tai chi and its self-defense techniques.

Q

Qi *See* Chi.

Qigong (chi gung, chi kung) Energy work/power. The ancient Chinese art and science of developing and cultivating chi by one's own effort. Qigong techniques may be done standing, moving, sitting, lying down and as partner exercises.

Qigong tui na (chi gung tui na, ch'i kung twei na) Therapeutic bodywork with chi. A specialty of Chinese medicine, where the healer directly emits and rebalances the chi in the patient's body to bring about a therapeutic result. Its diagnostic techniques are based on reading the energy of the external aura, as well as the subtle energy of the three internal tantiens of the body.

R

Right channel One of the three primary energy lines of the body. *See* Left channel.

Rooting The technique of sinking body energy and rooting it into the earth. It is difficult to physically move a martial artist who has mastered rooting. In the internal martial arts, rooting gives a practitioner tremendous power.

Rou Shou Soft Hands; also known as San Shou or Free Hands in Taiwan. A two-person fighting preparation technique practiced in bagua (and some hsing-i schools) in which the arms of the partners are in continuous spiraling contact. Rou Shou can be likened to a combination of tai chi Push Hands, judo and Wing Chun sticky hands.

S

Samadhi A meditative experience that is indicative of a specific stage of "enlightenment."

Single Palm Change (dan huan zhang, tan huan chang) The most fundamental technique in bagua. The Single Palm Change is a microcosm of the whole system based on the first (heaven) trigram of the *I Ching*.

Sixty-four hexagrams Sixty-four basic energetic changes of the *I Ching*.

Standing qigong (jan chuang, zhan zhuang) Qigong that is done standing still, either with the practioner's arms resting at the sides of the body or else held in the air in a static arm posture. Standing qigong is one of the most basic techniques for developing internal power.

Sun style tai chi A combination style of tai chi created by Sun Lu Tang that amalgamates the Hao style with hsing-i and bagua.

Synovial fluid A bodily fluid that is present in the space between the joints of the body.

T

Tae kwon do A Korean external martial art that emphasizes kicking techniques; also known as Korean karate.

Tai chi chuan (tai ji quan, taijiquan, tai chi ch'uan) Supreme ultimate martial arts fist. One of the three internal martial arts of China, most known for its emphasis on softness, slow-motion movement, and its sophisticated qigong methodology based on whole-body physical coordination. Done by the majority of its practitioners primarily for health, not combat. As a martial art, tai chi emphasizes softness, yielding techniques and counterattack strategies, and a blending of soft and hard internal power.

Tai Chi Classics A nineteenth-century treatise on the foundational principles of tai chi chuan, said to be written by Wang Tsung Yueh. Contains short, cryptic phrases having multilayered meanings.

Tang ni bu (t'ang ni pu) Mud-walking. The basic chi and physical mechanics principles upon which the Circle Walking steps of bagua are based.

Tantien (tant'ien, dantian) The three primary centers in the human body where chi collects, disperses and recirculates. They govern the energetic anatomy of a person. The practices of the three tantiens are at the operational root of all Chinese chi practices.

Tao/Taoism (dao) The Way. The practical mystical religion of China that forms the original underpinnings of classical Chinese culture, including the yin-yang play of opposites, Chinese medicine, and the art of strategy and war.

Tao Jia (dao jia, tao chia) The mystical inner esoteric practices of Taoism. Includes the beginning stage of Taoist meditation that involves methods for completely stilling the mind and an advanced stage, which involves internal alchemy, or transformation of inner energies for realizing and becoming one with the Tao, the nature of the universe itself.

Tao Jiao (dao jiao, tao chiao) The outer aspects of Taoism, including mediums, idol worship and fortune-telling.

Taoist master An accomplished or "enlightened" adept of Taoist meditation, who has reached and completed the highest practices in Taoism. These individuals are exceedingly rare.

Three burners (san jiao) A tenet of Chinese medicine concerning how the chi of the body is separated into three parts that need to be integrated to achieve optimum health and balanced chi circulation. The upper burner refers to the part of the body that includes the chest, arms, upper spine, neck and head. The middle burner begins at the solar plexus and ends at the lower tantien. It includes the middle spine, liver, kidneys and spleen. The lower burner includes the lower belly, lower spine, sexual organs, hips and legs.

Toe-out/toe-in (bai bu/kou bu) Basic step performed in Bagua Circle Walking.

Traditional Chinese martial arts The martial arts that traditionally existed in China before the Communist revolution. Traditional martial arts are based on pragmatic fighting skills with the religious and philosophical underpinnings of Confucian, Buddhist and Taoist precepts.

Tui na (tuina,twei na) The therapeutic bodywork system of China, which is considered to be of a higher level than ordinary Chinese massage (known as ammo). Included within its therapeutic interventions are acupressure, bonesetting, and joint and vertebral manipulations, along with deep tissue myofascial, craniosacral, tendon and ligament work, and internal organ/gland realignment and rebalancing. When combined therapeutically with qigong, it is called qigong tui na.

U

Universal Consciousness The underlying something, which cannot be defined, of which the whole universe is composed. Called the Tao in ancient China.

Upper tantien (dantian) Located in the brain, this tantien controls human perceptual mechanisms and psychic functions.

W

Wai ba jang (wai ba zhang, wai pa chang) Outer eight palms. Basic pre-birth bagua zhang practice of secondary circle-walking techniques that function as fighting applications only.

Water Element In Chinese cosmology, one of the basic energies or elements from which all manifested phenomena are created.

Water method A meditation or energetic technique that emphasizes using full effort without strain or force.

Wei chi The layer of energy between a person's skin and muscle that protects against disease entering the body from the external environment.

Wood Element In Chinese cosmology, one of the basic energies or elements from which all manifested phenomena are created.

Wu style tai chi A style of tai chi chuan especially known for its healing and meditation components. A small-frame fighting style that developed from the Yang style. Wu style is the second most popular form of tai chi in China and is becoming more available in the West.

Wu wei Doing without doing. The fundamental Taoist concept of having action arise from an empty mind without preconception or agenda, action that operates by simply following the natural course of universal energy as it manifests itself without strain or ego involvement.

Y

Yang style tai chi The most popular form of tai chi today.

Yin and yang meridans The twelve major vertical subtle energy channels of the body.

Yin-yang The classic Taoist concept that the universe is composed of opposites (sun/moon, active/passive, work/rest, happiness/sadness, etc.) that are not antagonistic, but complementary and necessary to fulfill each other. It is through the yin-yang play of opposites that all manifestation, obvious or subtle, occurs.

Z

Zen (Zen is Japanese; in Chinese: Chan) A spiritual discipline created by a fusion of Taoist and Buddhist methods. Zen practices are sometimes adapted to the martial arts. *See* Buddhism.

APPENDIX G

Taoism: A Living Tradition

Many traditions that are based on ancient philosophies and religions have vibrantly continued into modern times. Because they manifest in our lives today, they are called living traditions. These include Christianity, Islam, Judaism, Buddhism, yoga and Taoism. The latter three actively practice physical exercises and energy work.

Taoism is the least known of the living traditions. Although its main literary works—the *I Ching*, the writings of Chuang Tse and the *Tao Te Ching* by Lao Tse—are well known and available in many translations, the practical methods and techniques of implementing Taoist philosophy in daily life are little documented in the West.

One branch of living Taoist philosophy is about developing and using your personal chi or life-force energy to strengthen, heal and benefit yourself and others. This branch encompasses two broad traditions: Water and Fire. The Water tradition, based on the philosophies of Lao Tse, emphasizes effort without force, relaxation and letting go, as a flow of water slowly erodes rock. The Fire tradition, developed 1,500 years later, emphasizes force, pushing forward and breaking through barriers.

The Taoist lineages that Bruce Frantzis holds are in the Water tradition, which has received little exposure in the West. Part of his lineage empowers and directs him to bring practices based on that tradition to Westerners. He learned the Chinese language and became immersed in the traditions of China during his training there.

While Frantzis studied with his main teacher, Grandmaster Liu Hung Chieh, texts were presented as: "This is what they say; this is what they mean; this is how to do them." Frantzis offers an unprecedented bridge to this pragmatic approach to spirituality; in fact, we are not aware of any other English or European language source for this style of teaching. It means that spirituality is not just an aspiration for which people strive in the dark—"in a mirror, darkly,"—to quote St. Paul, but it can become a genuine, accomplishable reality.

The Frantzis Energy Arts System

Drawing on sixteen years of training in Asia, Bruce Frantzis has developed a practical, comprehensive system of programs that can enable people of all ages and fitness levels to increase their core energy and attain vibrant health.

Core Qigong Practices

The Frantzis Energy Arts® System includes six primary qigong courses that, together with the Longevity Breathing® program, progressively and safely incorporate all the aspects of neigong—the original chi cultivation (qigong) system in China that originated from the Taoists. Although the qigong techniques are very old, Bruce Frantzis' system of teaching them is unique. It is specifically tailored to Westerners and the needs of modern life. A good analogy is that Frantzis has created the cup—the Frantzis Energy Arts System—that can hold the wine—these ancient Taoist practices.

The core practices consist of:
- Taoist Longevity Breathing®
- Dragon and Tiger Medical Qigong
- Opening the Energy Gates of Your Body™ Qigong
- The Marriage of Heaven and Earth™ Qigong
- Bend the Bow Spinal™ Qigong
- Spiraling Energy Body™ Qigong
- Gods Playing in the Clouds™ Qigong

The core qigong programs were deliberately chosen because they are among the oldest, most effective and most treasured of Taoist energy practices. They are ideal for progressively incorporating the major components of neigong in a manner that is comprehensible and understandable to Westerners. They provide students with the foundation necessary for clearly and systematically learning and advancing their practice in Taoist energy arts.

Taoist Longevity Breathing

Frantzis has developed this method to teach authentic Taoist breathing in systematic stages. Breathing with the whole body has been used for millennia to enhance the ability to dissolve and release energy blockages in the mind/body, enhancing well-being and spiritual awareness. Incorporating these breathing techniques into any other Taoist energy practice will help bring out its full potential.

Dragon and Tiger Medical Qigong

This is one of the most direct and accessible low-impact qigong healing methods that China has produced. This 1,500-year-old form of medical qigong affects the human body in a manner similar to acupuncture. Its seven simple movements can be done by virtually anyone, whatever their age or state of health.

Opening the Energy Gates of Your Body Qigong

This program introduces 3,000-year-old qigong techniques that are fundamental to advancing any energy arts practice. Core exercises teach you the basic body alignments and how to increase your internal awareness of chi in your body and dissolve blocked energy.

The Marriage of Heaven and Earth Qigong

This qigong set incorporates techniques widely used in China to help heal back, neck, spine and joint problems. It is especially effective for helping to mitigate repetitive stress injury and carpal tunnel problems. This program teaches some important neigong components, including openings and closings (pulsing), more complex breathing techniques and how to move chi through the energy channels of the body.

Bend the Bow Spinal Qigong

Bend the Bow Spinal Qigong continues the work of strengthening and regenerating the spine that is learned in Marriage of Heaven and Earth Qigong. This program incorporates neigong components for awakening and controlling the energies of the spine.

Spiraling Energy Body Qigong

This advanced program teaches you to dramatically raise your energy level and master how energy moves in circles and spirals throughout your body. It incorporates neigong components for: directing the upward flow of energy; projecting chi along the body's spiraling pathways; delivering or projecting energy at will to or from any part of the body; and activating the body's left, right and central channels, and the microcosmic orbit.

Gods Playing in the Clouds Qigong

This qigong set incorporates some of the oldest and most powerful Taoist rejuvenation techniques. This program amplifies all the physical, breathing and energetic components learned in earlier qigong programs and completes the process of integrating all the components of neigong. It is also the final stage of learning to strengthen and balance the energies of your three tantiens, central energy channel and spine. Gods Playing in the Clouds Qigong serves as a spiritual bridge to Taoist meditation.

Taoist Longevity Yoga

Taoist yoga is ancient China's soft yet powerful alternative to what is popularly known today as Hatha yoga. The system Frantzis has developed to teach this is called Taoist Longevity Yoga.™ Its primary emphasis is to stimulate the flow of chi and free up any blocked energy. Combining gentle postures and Longevity Breathing techniques systematically opens the body's energy channels, thereby activating and stimulating chi flow. Postures are held from two to five minutes and require virtually no muscular effort, enabling you to easily focus on what is internal so you can feel where the chi is blocked and gently free it up.

Healing Others with Qigong Tui Na

Part of Frantzis' Taoist training was to become a Chinese doctor, primarily using the qigong healing techniques known as *qigong tui na*. During this training period, he worked with more than 10,000 patients. Frantzis no longer works as a qigong doctor, either privately or in clinics, but occasionally offers training in therapeutic healing techniques.

Qigong tui na is a special branch of Chinese medicine that is designed to unblock, free and balance chi in others. You learn to project energy from your hands, voice and eyes to facilitate healing using 200 hand techniques. You also learn how to avoid burnout from your therapeutic practice. To heal others, you must first learn to unblock and free your own chi and to control the specific pathways through which it flows.

Shengong

Whereas *chi* (or *qi*) means "energy," *shen* means "spirit." Spirit equals meditation, which equals spirituality. So the term *shengong* literally means "spirit work."

Chi practices can make your body healthier and physically stronger. Meditation is about going beyond the energy of your flesh and internal organs where the primal or instinctual emotions reside. In terms of meditation, shengong is the fusion of qigong with the emotional, mental, psychic and karmic energy bodies to the level of your essence. This is the point at which you move into Taoist meditation.

Taoist Meditation

Frantzis is a lineage holder in the gentle Water method of Taoist meditation passed down from the teachings of Lao Tse over 2,500 years ago. Taoist meditation is little known in the West and is often confused with Buddhism. In Taoism, the road to spirituality involves more than having health, calmness and a stable, peaceful mind. These are just the necessary prerequisites and are achieved through qigong, Longevity Breathing, tai chi and other Taoist energy programs.

Taoist meditation includes using chi to help you release anxieties, expectations, and negative emotions—referred to as blockages—that prevent you from feeling truly alive and joyful. The first goal is to address spiritual responsibility for yourself, helping you become a relaxed, spontaneous, fully mature and open human being. A second goal is awakening the great human potential inside you, fostering compassion and balance. The third is reaching inner stillness—a place deep inside you that is absolutely permanent and stable. As your practice deepens, the sixteen-part neigong system is brought into play to accelerate the evolutionary spiritual process.

Tai Chi and Bagua as Health and Meditation Arts

Tai chi and bagua practiced as health arts intensify the benefits of the core qigong practices.

Most Westerners learn tai chi purely as a health exercise rather than a martial art. Like all qigong programs, tai chi relaxes and regulates the central nervous system, releasing physical and emotional stress, and promoting mental and emotional well-being. Tai chi's gentle, non-jarring movements are ideal for people of any age and body type and can give them a high degree of relaxation, balance and physical coordination.

Tai chi is commonly referred to as moving meditation. Tai chi's slow, graceful movements provide relaxed focus, quiet down your internal dialogue and engender a deep sense of relaxation that helps release inner tensions. Only a few tai chi masters know how to transform the practice of tai chi to a complete Taoist moving meditation. Liu Hung Chieh taught Frantzis this tradition and empowered him to teach it.

Even more ancient than tai chi, the Circle Walking techniques of bagua were developed over 4,000 years ago in Taoist monasteries as a health and meditation art. The aim of these techniques is to open up the possibilities of the mind and achieve stillness and clarity; to generate a strong, healthy, disease-free body; and, perhaps more importantly, to maintain internal balance while either your inner world or the events of the external world are rapidly changing.

Tai Chi, Bagua and Hsing-i as Internal Martial Arts

The internal martial arts teach you to use relaxation, chi, and stillness of mind to accomplish the pragmatic goal of winning in a violent confrontation, rather than using muscular tension or anger for power.

Tai Chi Chuan

Tai chi is a potent martial art. Frantzis trained extensively in the traditional Wu, Yang and Chen styles of tai chi chuan, including short and long forms, Push Hands, self-defense techniques and such traditional weapons as sticks and swords.

Bagua Zhang

Bagua was designed to fight up to eight opponents at once. Virtually no other martial art system or style, internal or external, has combined and seamlessly integrated into one package the whole pantheon of martial arts fighting techniques as effectively as bagua.

Bagua is first and foremost an art of internal energy movement that embodies the eight primal energies that are encompassed by the eight trigrams of the *I Ching*. The basic internal power training consists of learning eight palm changes and combining them with walking, spiraling and twisting arm movements and constant changes of direction.

Hsing-i Chuan

Hsing-i (also transliterated as xing yi) emphasizes all aspects of the mind to create its forms and fighting movements. This art is an equally potent healing practice because it makes people healthy and then very strong.

Its five basic movements are related to the five primal elements or phases of energy—Metal, Water, Wood, Fire and Earth—upon which Chinese medicine is based and from which all manifested phenomena are created. Hsing-i's training is based on a linear, militaristic approach: marching in straight lines, with a powerful emphasis at the end of every technique on mentally or physically taking an enemy down.

Living Taoism Collection

The purpose of Bruce Frantzis' Living Taoism™ Collection is not to repeat or interpret ancient texts, but rather to show how Taoist practices are alive and extremely relevant to modern life. As personal health and energy systems, they can benefit you profoundly.

Books

Books in the Living Taoism Collection include
- *Opening the Energy Gates of Your Body: Qigong for Lifelong Health* (poster available)
- *Dragon and Tiger Medical Qigong: Health and Energy in Seven Simple Movements* (two-DVD set and poster available)
- *Tai Chi: Health for Life*
- *Chi Revolution,* which describes how chi is the power behind spirituality, meditation, sexual vitality, acupuncture, internal martial arts and the divination methods of the *I Ching*
- *The Power of Martial Arts and Chi: Combat and Energy Secrets of Bagua, Tai Chi and Hsing-i*

- Two volumes on the Water method of Taoist meditation, *Relaxing into Your Being: Chi, Breathing and Dissolving Inner Pain* and *The Great Stillness: Body Awareness, Moving Meditation and Sex Chi Gung (Qigong)*
- Frantzis' latest meditation book, *Tao of Letting Go: Meditation for Modern Living,* a companion to the CD-set described in the next section.

CDs and DVDs

DVD titles range from a general introduction to Taoist practices, *Taoist Energy Arts,* to specific instructional programs, such as Dragon and Tiger Qigong and Longevity Breathing. Audio programs available include the following:

- *Tao of Letting Go,* a six-CD set, reveals how the Inner Dissolving method of Taoist meditation can help you let go of tension, fear, anger and pain. Frantzis guides you through turning inward so that you can begin awakening your potential and move toward feeling more alive and joyful.
- *Ancient Songs of the Tao,* a three-CD set, is a collection of never-before-recorded chants in ancient Chinese. These Taoist liturgies are used to balance and transform the energetic frequencies within a human being.
- *Strings of the Tao,* in which Frantzis chants powerful liturgies accompanied by Kitaro violinist Steve Kindler.
- Taoist exercises for better sex, vibrant health and longevity are described in the two-CD set, *Chi Gung (Qigong) for the Sexes.*

Training Opportunities

Bruce Frantzis is the founder of Energy Arts, Inc. Energy Arts offers instructor certification programs, retreats, corporate and public workshops, and lectures worldwide. Frantzis teaches Energy Arts courses in qigong; Longevity Breathing; the internal martial arts of bagua, tai chi and hsing-i; Longevity Breathing Yoga; the healing techniques of qigong tui na; and the Water method of Taoist meditation.

Comprehensive multimedia training courses may also be available from time to time. Topics may include meditation, bagua, tai chi and qigong. See *EnergyArts.com* for current programs.

Instructor Certification

Prior training in Frantzis Energy Arts programs is a requirement for most instructor courses. The certification process is rigorous to ensure that instructors teach the authentic traditions inherent in these arts.

Train with a Frantzis Energy Arts Certified Instructor

The Energy Arts website, *EnergyArts.com,* contains a directory of all the certified instructors worldwide. Since Bruce Frantzis no longer offers regular ongoing classes, he recommends locating an instructor in your area for regular training and for building on or preparing for his teachings.

Contact Information

Energy Arts, Inc.
P.O. Box 99
Fairfax, CA 94978-0099
USA
Phone: (415) 454-5243

Visit EnergyArts.com:

- Join our list to get free articles and audio material by Bruce Frantzis.
- Receive the latest details on events and training materials.
- See video clips of qigong and martial arts forms.
- Find a Certified Energy Arts Instructor near you or learn how to become one.
- Inquire about hosting a workshop or speaking engagement.

Read Bruce's personal blog at **TaiChiMaster.com.**

BIBLIOGRAPHY

Capra, Fritjof, *The Tao of Physics*, Shambhala Publications, 2000.

Chuang Tzu, *The Way of Chuang Tzu*, Shambhala Publications, 2004, translated by Thomas Merton.

Lao Tse (Lao Tzu, Laozi), *Tao Te Ching*, various English translations available.

The Original I Ching Oracle, Watkins Publishing, 2005, translated by Rudolf Ritsema and Shantena Augusto Sabbadini.

Zhuangzi (Chuang Tzu), *Zhuangzi: Basic Writings*, Columbia University Press, 2003, translated by Burton Watson.

Zukav, Gary, *The Dancing Wu Li Masters*, HarperOne, 2001.